SURGICAL TECHNOLOGIST

SURGICAL TECHNOLOGIST

EXAMINATION REVIEW

THIRD EDITION

691 MULTIPLE CHOICE QUESTIONS AND REFERENCED EXPLANATORY ANSWERS

Norma C. Allen, R.N., M.S.
Instructor, Department of Surgical Services
New England Deaconess Hospital
Boston, Massachusetts

Diane Gulczynski, R.N., B.S.
Nurse Manager, Operating Room/Recovery Room
Faulkner Hospital
Jamaica Plain, Massachusetts

MEDICAL EXAMINATION PUBLISHING COMPANY

Allen, Norma C.
Surgical technologist examination review.

Bibliography: p.
1. Surgical technology—Examinations, questions, etc.
I. Gulczynski, Diane. II. Title. [DNLM: 1. Operating room Technicians—examination questions. 2. Surgical Nursing—examination questions. WY 18 A428s]
RD32.3.A445 1984 617'.9'076 84-14816
ISBN 0-87488-651-1

MEDICAL EXAMINATION PUBLISHING COMPANY
A Division of Elsevier Science Publishing Co., Inc.
52 Vanderbilt Avenue
New York, New York 10017

Printed in the United States of America

Contents

Preface

This volume is offered as an aid in self-assessment of operating room technologists who wish to assure themselves that their knowledge of technical preparation and assistance in surgical procedures is current and complete. It should allow the reader to recognize areas of weakness and provide an opportunity to broaden knowledge in the field of operating room technology.

Answers and a brief explanation, in addition to the references, are given for each multiple choice question. The reader is encouraged to consult this reference for more complete information.

About the Authors

NORMA ALLEN, R. N., M. S., C. N. O. R., is an Instructor for the Department of Surgical Services, New England Deaconess Hospital, Boston, Massachusetts.

Ms. Allen is a graduate of Arnot-Ogden Memorial Hospital School of Nursing, Elmira, New York. She received a Bachelor of Science Degree in Psychology/Rehabilitation Counseling from Emmanuel College, Boston, Massachusetts and a Master of Science Degree in Management from Lesley College, Cambridge, Massachusetts. Ms. Allen is a member of, and certified by, the Association of Operating Room Nurses and currently teaches a Postgraduate Program in Operating Room Nursing.

DIANE GULCZYNSKI, R. N., B. S., C. N. O. R., is the Nurse Manager of the Operating Room and Recovery Room, Faulkner Hospital, Jamaica Plain, Massachusetts. Ms. Gulczynski is a graduate of the New England Deaconess Hospital School of Nursing, Boston, Massachusetts. She received a Bachelor of Science Degree in Organizational Behavior from Lesley College, Cambridge, Massachusetts. Ms. Gulczynski is a member of, and certified by, the Association of Operating Room Nurses and is currently on the Board of Directors, Massachusetts Chapter I, Association of Operating Room Nurses.

Acknowledgments

A revision of a textbook can be a monumental task. The expertise of the original authors, Margaret A. Burns and Lois A. Morrissey, made our undertaking a less arduous one.

We also take this opportunity to express our appreciation to Margaret A. Burns for her support and direction in our nursing careers.

notice

The authors and the publisher of this book have made every effort to ensure that all therapeutic modalities that are recommended are in accordance with accepted standards at the time of publication.

The drugs specified within this book may not have specific approval by the Food and Drug Administration in regard to the indications and dosages that are recommended by the authors. The manufacturer's package insert is the best source of current prescribing information.

I

INTRODUCTION

1. INTRODUCTION

DIRECTIONS: Each of the questions or incomplete statements below is followed by five suggested answers or completions. Select the most appropriate answer(s).

---

1. An effective system of air conditioning and ventilation
   A. provides proper temperature and humidity to ensure the comfort of patient and staff
   B. reduces airborne bacteria
   C. maintains a temperature of 68-75° F and humidity at 50-55%
   D. produces a minimum of at least 25 changes of air per hour
   E. all of the above

2. Trans is a prefix meaning
   A. beyond, excessive
   B. across
   C. on the opposite side
   D. all
   E. around

3. The suffix itis means
   A. breaking down, cutting
   B. drawing, recording
   C. puncture, aspirate
   D. inflammation
   E. repair of

4. An infarct is
   A. an area of coagulation necrosis in a tissue due to lack of blood supply to a part
   B. the escape of abdominal contents through the site of an incision of a previous operation
   C. the same tension or concentration as blood
   D. a morbid tissue reaction due to injury or disease
   E. the process of becoming hard

5. The suffix <u>ectomy</u> means
   A. inflammation of
   B. surgical removal of dead tissue
   C. surgical removal
   D. abscess formation
   E. plastic repair

6. The suffix <u>ostomy</u> means
   A. plastic repair of tissue
   B. removal of cancerous lesion
   C. viewing of internal structures
   D. creating an artificial opening
   E. none of the above

7. Ischemic means
   A. air in the tissue
   B. delay of impulse
   C. localized anemia due to obstructive circulation
   D. a clot formed within a vessel
   E. spindle-shaped dilation of an artery

8. Abduction means
   A. rotation around an axis
   B. extension of the lower limb
   C. movement away from the midline
   D. movement toward the midline
   E. flexion and extension of the upper extremity

9. Hospitals must meet certain standards and are inspected periodically for licensure and accreditation. This is done by
   A. written reports
   B. on-site visit by state public health officials
   C. on-site visits by Joint Commission on Hospital Accreditation inspectors
   D. surveys done by the hospital administration
   E. none of the above

II

BASIC SCIENCES

2. ANATOMY AND PHYSIOLOGY

DIRECTIONS: Each of the questions or incomplete statements below is followed by a list of suggested answers or completions. Select the most appropriate answer(s).

A. Anatomy

10. A transverse plane is a line which divides the body into
    A. specific right angles
    B. two equal halves from the top of the head and between the knees and feet
    C. right and left sides
    D. upper and lower portions
    E. anterior and posterior halves

11. Metabolism is the
    A. ability to acquire, store, and use food for growth and repair, release of energy, and excretion of waste
    B. ability to acquire and use food
    C. ability to release energy and excrete waste
    D. ability to excrete waste or break down food only
    E. none of the above

12. Connective tissue forms the supporting structures of the body, binds and holds the structures in place, and also replaces dead cells. Which of the following could be classified as connective tissue?
    A. Adipose tissue
    B. Cartilage
    C. Fibrous tissue
    D. Areolar tissue
    E. All of the above

13. An articulation is a
    A. ligament
    B. union between two or more adjacent bones
    C. special name for a long bone
    D. cartilage
    E. muscle

14. The definition of arthritis is
    A. a fused joint
    B. an inflammation of a joint
    C. a disarticulation of a joint
    D. deposits of uric acid crystals in the joint
    E. a lack of synovial fluid

B. <u>Muscular/Skeletal System</u>

15. The bone at the posterior position of the skull is known as the
    A. parietal
    B. occipital
    C. temporal
    D. mastoid
    E. frontal

16. Skeletal muscles execute movements initiated by the will and are known as
    A. voluntary
    B. striated
    C. nonstriated
    D. smooth
    E. fascia

17. A joint is surrounded by a capsule of thin tissue filled with which of the following substances which serves to lubricate the cartilage?
    A. Protoplasm
    B. Synovial fluid
    C. Pericardial fluid
    D. Spinal fluid
    E. None of the above

18. Metacarpophalangeal and interphalangeal joints are examples of which of the following types of joints?
    A. Saddle
    B. Synovial
    C. Hinge
    D. Ball and socket
    E. None of the above

19. Extension is the
    A. opposite of flexion
    B. moving away from the central axis
    C. movement that reduces the angle of two movably articulated bones
    D. movement that increases the angle of two movably articulated bones
    E. none of the above

20. Protraction is the
    A. opposite of extraction
    B. outward protrusion of a body part
    C. turning in of a body part
    D. pivoting of a body part
    E. none of the above

21. The elbow represents a joint between the two forearm bones and the single upper arm bone, the
    A. radius
    B. fibula
    C. humerus
    D. ulna
    E. none of the above

22. The main shaft of the long bone is called the
    A. endosteum
    B. metaphysis
    C. diaphysis
    D. periosteum
    E. none of the above

23. Bone-forming cells are called
    A. nucleoblasts
    B. osteoblasts
    C. apetites
    D. tropocollagens
    E. none of the above

24. Osteoporosis
    A. is a weakening of the skeleton due to loss of minerals
    B. is found only in flat bones
    C. is likely to be caused by a hormone deficiency
    D. has a high incidence in postmenopausal females
    E. none of the above

25. Which of the following are specialized skeletal structures that generally transmit muscular pull to bones?
    A. Ligaments
    B. Tendons
    C. Fibers
    D. Connective tissue
    E. None of the above

26. Cartilage consists of
    A. hyaline
    B. elastic fibers
    C. inelastic fibers
    D. perichondrium
    E. all of the above

27. A typical bone is surrounded by
    A. periosteal membrane
    B. cancellous bone and marrow
    C. ligaments and tendons
    D. collagen fibers
    E. none of the above

28. Arthritis
    A. is a whimsical disease with spontaneous remission of symptoms
    B. is an inflammation of the synovial cavity
    C. occurs at any age, including childhood
    D. can be controlled by anti-inflammatory medications
    E. all of the above

29. The purpose of immobilization of a fracture is to
    A. hold bone fragments in contact with each other until healing takes place
    B. restrict activity of a part
    C. provide protection to the injured area
    D. prevent further nonunion of a fracture
    E. all of the above

30. Internal fixation of a long bone is achieved by using which of the following?
    A. Metal pins
    B. Intramedullary rods
    C. Compression plates
    D. Nails
    E. All of the above

31. A halo cast is used to immobilize
    A. a lumbar dislocation
    B. a cervical fracture
    C. the cervical spine following cervical spinal fusion
    D. all types of fusions to prevent displacement of bone grafts
    E. all of the above

32. The layer of connective tissue which covers muscle tissue is known as
    A. tendon
    B. endomysium
    C. fascia
    D. epimysium
    E. perimysium

33. A ganglion may be defined as
    A. a group of nerve cells outside the brain and spinal cord
    B. the interlacing of an axon and dendrites
    C. a "bump"
    D. nerve endings
    E. none of the above

C. Nervous System

34. The brain and spinal cord are enclosed by three membranes. The membrane which lies proximal to the cranium is the (outside)
    A. dura mater
    B. pia mater
    C. arachnoid mater
    D. mater
    E. subdural mater

35. The three layers of tissue which cover and protect the brain and spinal cord are known as the meninges. The layer which lies in intimate contact with the brain is the
    A. duramater
    B. pia mater
    C. arachnoid mater
    D. subarachnoid mater
    E. none of the above

36. Cerebrospinal fluid is found circulating
    A. in the subdural space
    B. in the subarachnoid space
    C. in the subapical space
    D. only in the ventricles of the brain
    E. only through the convolutions of the brain

37. The brain is composed of five fairly distinct components. The largest part of the brain is the
    A. cerebrum
    B. pons
    C. midbrain
    D. cerebellum
    E. medulla oblongata

38. Which of the following is the function of the spinal cord?
    A. An important center of reflex action—body and limbs
    B. Principal conduction path to and from the higher centers in the cord and brain
    C. Afferent pathway
    D. Efferent pathway only
    E. Sympathetic chain

39. There are how many pairs of cranial nerves which originate from the undersurface of the brain and are classified as motor, sensory, and mixed nerves?
    A. 9
    B. 10
    C. 11
    D. 12
    E. 13

40. The two principal divisions of the nervous system are the
    A. peripheral nervous system
    B. autonomic nervous system
    C. parasympathetic nervous system
    D. central nervous system
    E. sympathetic nervous system

41. The peripheral nervous system is subdivided into
    A. somatic
    B. afferent
    C. efferent
    D. autonomic
    E. none of the above

42. Sympathetic nerves operate to
    A. stimulate organs
    B. mobilize energy
    C. conserve and restore energy
    D. slow heart rate
    E. all of the above

43. Which of the following are short, highly branched fibers specialized to receive neural impulses?
    A. Neurofilaments
    B. Dendrites
    C. Axons
    D. Neurofibrils
    E. None of the above

44. Multiple sclerosis
    A. is a neurological disease
    B. causes patches of myelin to deteriorate
    C. interferes with conduction of neural impulses
    D. causes victims to suffer from loss of coordination
    E. all of the above

45. Reflex action is
    A. a single neural response in human beings
    B. our response to external stimuli
    C. protective in helping to maintain the integrity of the body
    D. a response to a specific stimulus
    E. all of the above

46. Another name for horse's tail is
    A. spinal cord
    B. cauda equina
    C. gray matter
    D. subdural space
    E. none of the above

47. The meninges consist of which of the following?
    A. Dura mater
    B. Epidural space
    C. Arachnoid
    D. Pia mater
    E. All of the above

48. The main functions of the spinal cord are to
    A. control reflex activities of the body
    B. transmit information back and forth to the brain
    C. convey voluntary motor impulses to spinal nerves
    D. influence movements related to posture
    E. all of the above

49. The hypothalamus
    A. is the most important output pathway and relay station between the cerebral cortex and lower autonomic centers
    B. is a link between the nervous and endocrine systems
    C. helps to maintain water balance
    D. regulates body temperature
    E. all of the above

50. Each hemisphere is divided into how many lobes?
    A. 4
    B. 5
    C. 6
    D. 8
    E. None of the above

51. The most anterior portion of each frontal lobe is known as the
    A. primary auditory area
    B. primary motor area
    C. prefrontal lobe
    D. central fissure
    E. none of the above

52. A disorder in which movement is shaky and difficult is known as
    A. Parkinson's disease
    B. von Willebrand's disease
    C. neuralgia
    D. neuropathy
    E. none of the above

53. How many pairs of cranial nerves emerge from the brain itself?
    A. 10
    B. 8
    C. 14
    D. 12
    E. None of the above

54. How many pairs of spinal nerves emerge from the spinal cord?
    A. 31
    B. 29
    C. 24
    D. 18
    E. None of the above

D. Digestive System

55. The structures and organs which lie in and along the alimentary canal form the digestive system. What occurs within the digestive tract?
    A. Food is moved through the tract and discarded
    B. Food is broken down, absorbed, and discarded
    C. Food is broken down physically and chemically, absorbed, and discarded
    D. Food is tasted, used for cells if necessary, and discarded
    E. Only food which contains protein is of any use and only that protein is used

56. There are three salivary glands that secrete saliva, which softens food. The names of these glands are parotid and
    A. submaxillary, submandibular
    B. submandibular, sublingual
    C. submarillary, sublingual
    D. maxillary, frontal
    E. frontal, sublingual

57. The function of the pharynx is to
   A. act as a passageway for air and as a resonating cavity for voice production
   B. act as a resonating cavity for voice production
   C. begin the process of digestion
   D. act as a passageway for food
   E. act as a passageway for air and food and as a resonating cavity for voice production

58. The esophagus is a muscular tube which begins at the lower end of the pharynx and terminates in the upper end of the stomach. Another name for the esophagus is the
   A. gullet
   B. buccal cavity
   C. pharyngeal cavity
   D. gastropharyngeal tube
   E. none of the above

59. The stomach is divided into multiple portions. The portion which surrounds the esophageal opening is the
   A. pylorus
   B. fundus
   C. body
   D. antrum
   E. cardia

60. The rounded-tip portion of the stomach is known as the
   A. pylorus
   B. fundus
   C. body
   D. antrum
   E. cardia

61. For descriptive purposes, the small intestine is divided into portions. These are the
   A. duodenum, jejunum, and ileum
   B. pylorus, duodenum, and ileum
   C. duodenum, jejunum, and sigmoid
   D. pylorus and ileum
   E. duodenum and ileum

62. The constricted lower portion of the stomach is known as the
    A. pylorus
    B. fundus
    C. body
    D. antrum
    E. cardia

63. The functions of the small intestine are the
    A. digestion and absorption of food
    B. absorption of fats and carbohydrates
    C. production of fecal material and serving as a passageway for feces
    D. production of hormones necessary for the breakdown of food
    E. absorption of food and production of bile

64. The large intestine (colon) is divided into: ascending
    A. and descending
    B. transverse, descending
    C. descending, rectum
    D. transverse, descending, rectum
    E. transverse, descending, sigmoid

65. The accessory organs of digestion are the pancreas, liver, and gall bladder. The pancreas is divided into the head, body, and tail. The head of the pancreas is located
    A. by the spleen
    B. tucked under the left lobe of the liver
    C. tucked under the right lobe of the liver
    D. filling the curve of the duodenum
    E. enmeshed in the jejunum

66. The pancreatic duct (duct of Wirsung) and the common bile duct unite and form a dilated tube known as the
    A. Wirsung tube
    B. ampulla of Wirsung
    C. ampulla of Vater
    D. ampulla of Santorini
    E. ampulla of Oddi

67. The pancreas produces two secretions, pancreatic juice and insulin. The special cells which produce insulin are known as the
    A. islets of Langerhans
    B. islets of Banting
    C. alveoli
    D. islets of Vater
    E. islets of Santorini

68. The hepatic duct is the union of two main ducts from the right and left sides of the liver. The hepatic duct and which of the following ducts unite to form the common bile duct?
    A. Cystic
    B. Cholecystic
    C. Hepatic accessory
    D. Intralobular
    E. Celiac

69. The gall bladder is a pear-shaped sac found in the gall-bladder fossa on the undersurface of the liver. The main function of the gall bladder is
    A. the production of bile
    B. the storage of bile
    C. to act as a collection sac when an overproduction of bile is secreted
    D. no specific function
    E. to aid in the digestion of toxic substances

E. Blood

70. Hemolysis is defined as the
    A. overproduction of red blood cells
    B. destruction of red blood cells
    C. manufacturing of red blood cells
    D. breaking in half of red blood cells
    E. aggregation of red blood cells

71. Hematocrit is
    A. a special protein in the blood
    B. the volume of packed red cells
    C. a protective agent in the blood
    D. the volume of serum
    E. all enzyme which is present in the blood

72. Another name for white blood cells is
    A. lymphocytes
    B. monocytes
    C. eosinophils
    D. basophils
    E. leukocytes

73. Platelets are formed in red bone marrow. Their function is to
    A. carry oxygen
    B. carry carbon dioxide
    C. help in the protection against pathogenic bacteria
    D. assist in tissue repair
    E. assist in the clotting of blood

74. An embolism is
    A. a special factor necessary for the clotting of blood
    B. another name for a thrombus
    C. a stationary blood clot
    D. a travelling blood clot
    E. a condition of vitamin K deficiency

75. Polycythemia is a
    A. low hematocrit
    B. high hematocrit
    C. low white blood cell count
    D. high white blood cell count
    E. none of the above

76. Another name for red blood cells is
    A. leukocytes
    B. monocytes
    C. erythrocytes
    D. fibrinogen
    E. none of the above

77. A normal hemoglobin for women is
    A. 13-16 g/100 ml
    B. 14-17 g/100 ml
    C. 12-15 g/100 ml
    D. 10-12 g/100 ml
    E. none of the above

78. Which of the following is an insoluble fibrous protein that reinforces the platelet plug?
   A. Fibrin
   B. Thrombin
   C. Prothrombin
   D. Fibrinogen
   E. None of the above

79. Deficiencies in the number of platelets can produce which of the following disorders?
   A. Blood
   B. Factor VIII
   C. Clotting
   D. Hemolysis
   E. None of the above

80. A blood vessel that conducts blood away from the heart and to the organs and tissues is called
   A. a capillary
   B. an arteriole
   C. an artery
   D. a sinusoid
   E. none of the above

81. In the liver, spleen, and bone marrow, arterioles and venules are connected by passages known as
   A. ventricles
   B. precapillary sphincters
   C. sinusoids
   D. veins
   E. none of the above

82. Plasma contains what percentage of water?
   A. 85
   B. 73
   C. 100
   D. 92
   E. None of the above

83. A man weighing about 154 lb would have a blood volume of
   A. 5 qt
   B. 6 qt
   C. 7 qt
   D. 8 qt
   E. none of the above

84. Normal circulating blood volume is
   A. 6%
   B. 7%
   C. 8%
   D. 10%
   E. none of the above

F. <u>Cardiac</u>

85. The serous membrane which covers the heart is the
   A. pericardium
   B. epicardium
   C. myocardium
   D. endocardium
   E. carditis

86. The outside layer of the heart is the
   A. pericardium
   B. myocardium
   C. epicardium
   D. endocardium
   E. tunica media

87. Which of these two large veins brings deoxygenated blood to the right atrium?
   A. Inferior vena cava
   B. Superior vena cava
   C. Pulmonary artery
   D. Aorta
   E. External jugular vein

88. Between the right and left auricles and ventricles there are mechanical devices known as valves which allow blood flow into the ventricles as long as the pressure is higher in the auricles. The right atrioventricular valve is the
   A. biscuspid
   B. mitral
   C. tricuspid
   D. semilunar
   E. left semilunar

89. The sinoatrial (SA) node is the pacemaker of the heart. It is located
    A. in the septal wall
    B. in the left ventricle
    C. in the myocardium
    D. at the junction of the superior vena cava and right atrium
    E. at the junction of the pulmonary artery and right ventricle

90. The atrioventricular (AV) node is found in the lower portion of the inner wall of the right atrium. It acts as a relay station, picks up impulses, and sends them to the His bundle which has fibers through the ventricular system and causes
    A. auricles to relax
    B. ventricles to contract
    C. ventricles to dilate
    D. auricles to contract
    E. unknown

91. Diastole is defined as
    A. a period of contraction
    B. a period of relaxation
    C. what is monitored by a stethoscope
    D. what is monitored by a sphygmomanometer
    E. what is seen on an EKG monitor

92. A heart can go into atrial or ventricular fibrillation. Fibrillation is defined as a
    A. normal heart rate
    B. heart rate under 50
    C. normal heart rate
    D. rapid, irregular movement
    E. slow, irregular pulse rate

93. Tachycardia is defined as a
    A. heart rate over 100
    B. heart rate under 40
    C. normal heart rate
    D. rapid, irregular pulse rate
    E. slow, irregular pulse rate

94. Bradycardia is defined as a
   A. heart rate over 100
   B. heart rate under 40
   C. heart rate under 60
   D. rapid, irregular pulse rate
   E. slow, irregular pulse rate

95. Epinephrine and adrenaline affect the heart rate by
   A. increasing the frequency and force
   B. acting as vasoconstrictors
   C. decreasing the frequency and force
   D. acting as a vasodilator
   E. increasing frequency and decreasing force

G. Circulatory System

96. The superior and inferior mesenteric arteries supply what organs?
   A. Kidney
   B. Large and small intestines
   C. Diaphragm
   D. Stomach
   E. Pancreas

97. The descending aorta bifurcates at the fourth lumbar vertebra into
   A. internal and external iliacs
   B. femoral and saphenous
   C. two femorals
   D. two common iliacs
   E. two saphenous

98. The circle of Willis is found
   A. behind the knee
   B. at the base of the neck
   C. at the base of the brain
   D. in the axillary region
   E. in the inguinal region

99. The portal system is a group of veins which unite and carry blood to the liver. These veins come from which of the following organs?
   A. Stomach
   B. Pancreas
   C. Large and small intestines
   D. Kidneys
   E. Gallbladders

100. The coronary circulation consists of which of the following branches?
   A. Left coronary artery
   B. Right coronary artery
   C. Posterior descending branch
   D. Circumflex
   E. All of the above

101. The thoracic aorta supplies oxygenated blood to which of the following regions?
   A. Bronchi
   B. Esophagus
   C. Spleen
   D. Chest muscles
   E. None of the above

102. Pulmonary umbrellas are placed in the
   A. inferior vena cava
   B. superior vena cava
   C. external jugular
   D. brachiocephalic
   E. none of the above

103. The liver is supplied with oxygenated blood by the
   A. celiac artery
   B. supra renals
   C. hepatic artery
   D. inferior mesenteric artery
   E. none of the above

104. Pulmonary circulation consists of
   A. oxygenated blood returning to the heart for systemic circulation
   B. blood flowing into the extensive capillary networks in the walls of the air sacs
   C. two pulmonary veins which exit from each lung and conduct their load of oxygenated blood to the left atrium
   D. pulmonary arteries which transport deoxygenated blood
   E. all of the above

105. Blood is supplied to the esophagus from branches of the
   A. inferior thyroid
   B. thoracic aorta
   C. celiac arteries
   D. mesenteric artery
   E. none of the above

106. Blood supply to the ascending colon, hepatic flexure, and transverse colon comes from the
   A. superior mesenteric artery
   B. inferior mesenteric artery
   C. thoracic aorta
   D. celiac arteries
   E. none of the above

107. The blood supply of the kidney is conveyed through the
   A. thoracic aorta
   B. renal artery
   C. lobular arteries
   D. renal pelvis
   E. none of the above

108. Each fallopian tube receives its blood supply from the branches of the
   A. uterine arteries
   B. ovarian arteries
   C. inferior epigastric artery
   D. renal artery
   E. none of the above

H. Urinary System

109. On the concave border of the kidney is the hilum. What structures enter or leave the kidney at this point?
   A. Blood vessels and lymph vessels
   B. Ureter and blood vessels
   C. Ureter, blood vessels, lymph vessels, and nerves
   D. Ureter only
   E. Blood vessels only

110. The upper end of the ureter expands into a funnel-shaped cavity known as the pelvis of the kidney. What root word refers to kidney pelvis?
   A. Pyelo
   B. Pyloro
   C. Cysto
   D. Nephro
   E. Hydro

111. The function of the nephron is to
   A. manufacture urine
   B. filter the liquid portion of blood, remove liquid wastes, collect urine
   C. filter blood
   D. regulate sodium chloride content
   E. none of the above

112. Hematuria is
   A. pus in the urine
   B. albumin in the urine
   C. glucose in the urine
   D. blood in the urine
   E. none of the above

113. The calyces in the kidney unite and form a dilation which resembles a funnel and is known as the
   A. renal calyces
   B. renal pelvis
   C. renal calculi
   D. renal mucosal fold
   E. none of the above

114. Another name for the external urinary orifice of women is the
   A. meatus
   B. sphincter
   C. glans
   D. os
   E. trigone

115. The testes are two glandular organs located in the scrotum and suspended from the inguinal region by the spermatic cord. The spermatic cord contains the
   A. vas deferens
   B. vas deferens, spermatic artery and vein
   C. vas deferens and nerve fibers
   D. vas
   E. spermatic artery and vein, lymph vessels, and nerve fibers

116. The prostate gland is located
   A. surrounding the bladder
   B. posterior to the bladder
   C. inferior to the bladder and surrounding the first section of the urethra
   D. anterior to the bladder
   E. not considered a component part of the reproductive system

117. The accessory reproductive glands of men include the
   A. seminal vesicles
   B. prostate gland
   C. bulbourethral gland
   D. islets of Langerhans
   E. none of the above

118. The ureters and blood vessels are attached to the area of the concave edge called the
   A. renal pelvis
   B. hilum
   C. capsule
   D. trigone
   E. none of the above

119. The antidiuretic hormone (ADH) is secreted by the
   A. adrenal glands
   B. posterior pituitary gland
   C. hypothalamus
   D. kidneys
   E. none of the above

120. Polyuria is
   A. decreased urine output
   B. painful urination
   C. increased urine output of poor quality
   D. sugar diabetes
   E. none of the above

121. Renal failure may be caused by
   A. pyelonephritis
   B. glomerulonephritis
   C. acute tubular necrosis
   D. hydrocephalus
   E. none of the above

122. Gout is
   A. an extremely painful disease
   B. deposits of uric acid crystals
   C. commonly found in the joint cavities
   D. defective excretion of blood uric acid
   E. all of the above

123. What other organ in addition to the kidney has the ability to adjust and maintain hemostasis?
   A. Heart
   B. Gastric system
   C. Liver
   D. All of the above
   E. None of the above

124. Another word for urination is
   A. uremia
   B. anuria
   C. micturition
   D. polyuria
   E. none of the above

125. Which layer of the bladder is specially adapted to stretching?
   A. Outer serosa
   B. Detrusor muscle
   C. Transitional epithelium
   D. Mucosa
   E. None of the above

126. Which of the following actions on the ureters delivers urine into the bladder?
   A. Peristalsis
   B. Gravity
   C. Internal pressure of kidney build-up
   D. All of the above
   E. None of the above

I. Gynecology

127. The perineum is the muscular floor of the pelvis and is in the area between the
   - A. clitoris and urinary meatus
   - B. urinary meatus and vaginal orifice
   - C. vaginal orifice and anus
   - D. mons pubis and anus
   - E. none of the above

128. There are two ovaries, one at each side of the pelvis. The ovaries produce
   - A. ova only
   - B. estrogen
   - C. progesterone
   - D. ova and estrogen
   - E. ova, estrogen, and progesterone

129. What is an ectopic pregnancy?
   - A. Fertilized ovum implanted in fallopian tube
   - B. Fertilized ovum implanted in uterus
   - C. Fertilized ovum implanted in pelvic cavity
   - D. An unusually prolonged pregnancy which is terminated by cesarean section
   - E. A calcified embryo

130. The location of the uterus is
   - A. anterior to the urinary bladder
   - B. posterior to the urinary bladder
   - C. posterior to the rectum
   - D. anterior to the rectum and posterior to the urinary bladder
   - E. anterior to the symphysis pubis

131. The walls of the uterus are thick and have three layers. The external layer is known as the serous; the muscular layer is known as the
   - A. peritoneum
   - B. endometrium
   - C. myometrium
   - D. epicardium
   - E. myocardium

132. The breasts are accessory organs of the female reproductive system. The root word which refers to breasts is
    A. mast
    B. myo
    C. hept
    D. oophoro
    E. myringo

133. The ovaries produce ova and the female sex hormone called
    A. follicle-stimulating hormone (FSH)
    B. luteinizing hormone (LH)
    C. estrogen
    D. progesterone
    E. all of the above

134. The free end of the fallopian tube has long, fingerlike projections called
    A. oviducts
    B. fimbriae
    C. infundibulum
    D. Purkinje's fibers
    E. none of the above

135. Salpingitis is
    A. an inflammation of the uterus
    B. an inflammation of the uterine tubes
    C. often caused by gonorrheal infections
    D. often caused by syphilis
    E. none of the above

136. A tipped uterus is
    A. normal
    B. one that has shifted from the normal position
    C. a response to estrogen and progesterone from the ovary
    D. only treatable through surgical intervention
    E. none of the above

137. The endoscopic visualization of the peritoneal cavity through the anterior abdominal wall is referred to as a
    A. culdoscopy
    B. laparoscopy
    C. cystoscopy
    D. bronchoscopy
    E. none of the above

J. Respiratory

138. The larynx is composed of cartilage and has a protective structure at its superior portion. This structure prevents foreign material from entering the larynx. It is the
A. glottis
B. thyroid cartilage
C. epiglottis
D. cricoid cartilage
E. Adam's apple

139. The pleura is a transparent, thin, moist serous membrane which encloses each lung. The pleura has two layers. The portion which lies directly on the lung is the
A. parietal pleura
B. pulmonary pleura
C. visceral pleura
D. azygos pleura
E. none of the above

140. The mediastinum lies between the right and left pleurae in the middle of the chest and contains the
A. thymus
B. heart and great vessels
C. esophagus
D. trachea, lymph nodes, and vessels
E. all of the above

141. During inspiration, what occurs?
A. Intercostal muscles contract
B. Intercostal muscles relax
C. Diaphragm contracts and moves down to enlarge the thoracic cavity
D. inflation of pericardial sac
E. none of the above

142. The respiratory center is located in the
A. medulla and pons
B. lungs
C. cerebellum
D. cerebrum
E. pons only

143. The term which means difficult respiration is
   A. eupnea
   B. dyspnea
   C. apnea
   D. Cheyne-Stokes
   E. hyperpnea

144. The term which means lack of breathing is
   A. eupnea
   B. dyspnea
   C. apnea
   D. Cheyne-Stokes
   E. hyperpnea

145. Anoxia means
   A. absence of oxygen
   B. obstruction to the airway
   C. lack of breathing
   D. quiet respiration
   E. none of the above

146. One or more chest tubes may be used for postoperative closed chest drainage to provide
   A. a conduit for drainage of blood
   B. a conduit for fluid drainage from the intrapleural space
   C. reestablishment of a negative pressure in the intrapleural space
   D. none of the above
   E. all of the above

147. Endoscopic procedures pertinent to thoracic surgery are
   A. bronchoscopy
   B. esophagoscopy
   C. mediastinoscopy
   D. none of the above
   E. all of the above

148. Procedures involving the lungs are
   A. open and closed lung biopsies
   B. segmental resection
   C. wedge resection
   D. lobectomy
   E. all of the above

149. A talc povdraine is indicated for what physiological condition?
   A. Empyema
   B. Spontaneous pneumothorax
   C. Pleural effusions
   D. Emphysema
   E. None of the above

150. Pneumonectomy is the
   A. excision of one or more lobes of the lung
   B. excision of the entire lung
   C. same as an anterior thoracoplasty
   D. all of the above
   E. none of the above

K. Eye

151. The organ of vision is the eye, but also included in the visual apparatus one would have to include the
   A. temporal lobe of the cerebrum
   B. occipital lobe of the cerebrum
   C. optic nerve
   D. A and C
   E. B and C

152. Accessory organs of the eye are: eyebrows, eyelids, conjunctiva, muscles of the eye, lacrimal glands and ducts, and a special fascial tissue. The mucous membrane which lines the inner surface of the eyelid and covers the front portion of the eyeball is known as the
   A. conjunctiva
   B. sclera
   C. choroid
   D. retina
   E. cornea

153. The purpose of lacrimal secretions is to
   A. illustrate painful emotions
   B. keep the surface of the eyes moist and to help remove foreign bodies
   C. help remove microorganisms and dust
   D. all of the above
   E. B and C

154. The eyeball is composed of three layers of tissue. The outer layer is the
   A. sclera
   B. conjunctiva
   C. choroid
   D. retina
   E. vitreous humor

155. The cornea is
   A. transparent
   B. the window of the eye
   C. continuous with the sclera
   D. the pigmented area of the eye
   E. none of the above

156. The middle layer of the eyeball is the choroid, which contains the blood vessels that supply the eye. The colored portion of the choroid is the
   A. cornea
   B. pupil
   C. iris
   D. rods and cones
   E. retina

157. The function of the retina is to
   A. regulate the pressure in the anterior chamber or cavity
   B. receive and transmit images to the cerebrum
   C. receive and transmit images to the cerebellum
   D. regulate the pressure in the posterior chamber
   E. receive images in bright light only

158. The name of the nerve which carries sign impulses to the brain is the
   A. trochlear nerve
   B. trigeminal nerve
   C. oculomotor nerve
   D. optic nerve
   E. acoustic nerve

159. The point of the retina is of great importance and is known as the fovea centralis. Why is the fovea of such importance?
   A. It is directly concerned with the optic nerve
   B. It is the center of direct vision
   C. It is the refractive body
   D. It is the entry point of the optic nerve
   E. None of the above

160. A cataract could be described as
   A. an opaque lens
   B. a damaged cornea
   C. a detached retina
   D. a permanently constricted pupil
   E. none of the above

161. Dilating drops that are commonly used to dilate the pupils in order to examine the retina are
   A. mydriatics
   B. corticosteroids
   C. cycloplegics
   D. mistic drops
   E. none of the above

162. Which of the following is the inability to direct both eyes at the same object?
   A. Ectropion
   B. Chalgion
   C. Strabismus
   D. Cataract
   E. None of the above

163. Keratoplasty is
   A. the repair of the lower lid
   B. a corneal transplant
   C. the insertion of an intraocular lens
   D. a repair of a fracture of the orbit
   E. none of the above

164. The surgical procedure for glaucoma is
   A. Elliot trephination
   B. cyclodialysis
   C. iridectomy
   D. iridencleisis
   E. all of the above

165. Which of the following methods of cataract removal consists of removing the lens within its capsule?
   A. Intracapsular
   B. Extracapsular
   C. Cryoestractor
   D. Cauterization
   E. None of the above

L. Endocrine System

166. The endocrine system
   A. governs body processes such as growth and metabolism
   B. utilizes the bloodstream to distribute chemical messengers (hormones)
   C. functions closely with the nervous system to respond to environmental changes
   D. functions mainly in reproduction
   E. none of the above

167. Which of the following is a disorder of the pituitary gland?
   A. Giantism—occurs before skeletal maturity
   B. Acromegaly—excess growth after maturity
   C. Infantilism
   D. Diabetes insipidus—excessive dilute urine production
   E. All of the above

168. Hyperthyroidism (Graves' disease) is caused by overproduction of thyroxin due to thyroid tumor. Which of the following symptoms would be present?
   A. Excessive nervousness
   B. Weight loss
   C. Bulging of the eyes, exophthalmus
   D. Elevated heart rate and blood pressure
   E. All of the above

169. Simple goiter
   A. is often malignant
   B. is a result of insufficient dietary iodine
   C. is a dietary deficiency of iodine in a pregnant woman that may result in insufficient thyroxin production by the embryo; cretinism (idiocy) may occur
   D. can be treated, all but cretinism, by administering thyroid tablets
   E. none of the above

170. Calcium is important to the body for which of the following reasons?
   A. It is a structural component of bones and teeth
   B. Muscular contraction depends on calcium
   C. It is involved in nervous irritability
   D. It is involved in clotting of blood
   E. All of the above

171. The adrenal glands are composed of two parts, the outer layer or cortex and the inner layer or medulla. One of the hormones of the medulla which we hear a great deal about is
   A. epinephrine
   B. cortin
   C. ACTH
   D. aldosterone
   E. androgen

172. The hormone produced by the islets of Langerhans is
   A. adrenaline
   B. epinephrine
   C. insulin
   D. estrogen
   E. androgen

173. Electrolytes are
   A. substances which split into anions when placed in water
   B. classified as anions
   C. classified as cations
   D. all of the above
   E. A only

174. ADH helps the body
   A. to conserve water
   B. to regulate temperature control
   C. in the process of growth
   D. all of the above
   E. none of the above

175. Somatotropin is another name for
   A. the anterior pituitary gland
   B. the growth hormone
   C. the hypothalamus
   D. Addison's disease
   E. none of the above

176. Very small amounts of both androgens and estrogens are secreted in both sexes by which of the following?
   A. Pancreas
   B. Kidneys
   C. Adrenal cortex
   D. Pituitary gland
   E. None of the above

177. An adrenalectomy may be performed for which of the following?
   A. Neoplasm
   B. Hypersecretion
   C. Secondary treatments of neoplasm
   D. Benign enlargement
   E. None of the above

178. Cysts of the pancreas may be caused by
   A. congenital factors
   B. inflammation
   C. trauma
   D. parasites
   E. all of the above

3. MICROBIOLOGY

DIRECTIONS: Each of the questions or incomplete statements below is followed by five suggested answers or completions. Select the most appropriate answer(s).

---

179. Which of the following cocci type organisms is (are) normally found on the skin but can cause wound infections under certain conditions?
   - A. Diplococcus pneumoniae
   - B. Hemolytic streptococci
   - •C. Staphylococcus aureus
   - D. Bacillus botulinum
   - E. Hemophilus influenzae

180. Diplococcus pneumoniae causes
   - A. food poisoning
   - B. gonorrhea
   - C. syphilis
   - D. skin infection
   - •E. none of the above

181. Clostridium welchii causes
   - •A. gas gangrene
   - B. anthrax
   - C. athlete's foot
   - D. dysentery
   - E. urinary tract infections

182. The normal flora (organisms) found in the human intestinal tract are
   - •A. Escherichia coli
   - B. Cornyebacterium diphtheriae
   - C. Mycobacterium tuberculosis
   - D. Clostridium welchii
   - E. Clostridium perfringens

183. Which of the following organisms is (are) found in contaminated water, milk, and eggs and may cause gastroenteritis?
   A. Proteus
   B. Pseudomonas
   • C. Salmonella
   D. Coli
   E. Aerobacter aerogens

184. The causative organism of syphilis is
   A. Trichophyton mentagrophytes
   • B. Treponema pallidum
   C. Candida albicans
   D. Pseudomonas
   E. E. coli

185. There are numerous disease processes associated with Staphylococcus aureus. Which of the following are portals of entry?
   • A. Skin
   • B. Respiratory tract
   • C. Genitourinary
   D. Gastrointestinal
   E. All of the above

186. The first infection that develops after microbial invasion is
   A. secondary
   • B. systemic
   C. sepsis
   D. primary
   E. none of the above

187. Which of the following are microorganisms which habitually live in the epidermis?
   A. Transient
   •B. Resident
   C. Endotoxin
   D. Hospital acquired
   E. None of the above

188. Which of the following usually gains entrance to the tissues after being deposited on and by burrowing through mucous membrane?
   A. E. coli
   B. Pseudomonas
   •C. N. gonorrhoeae
   D. Salmonella
   E. None of the above

189. Prevention of streptococcal infection can be accomplished by
   .A. adherence to aseptic techniques
   .B. proper handling of contaminated clothing and masks
   •C. adequate ventilation
   D. none of the above
   E. all of the above

4. PHYSIOLOGY OF INJURY AND WOUND HEALING

DIRECTIONS: Each of the questions or incomplete statements below is followed by five suggested answers or completions. Select the most appropriate answer(s).

---

190. Evisceration may be defined as
    A. bodily injury produced by violence
    B. abdominal viscera of the human body
    • C. breakdown of a suture line and protrusion of abdominal viscera
    D. formation of new tissue
    E. rectal prolapse

191. The defense mechanism of the body's local tissues to any irritating or injurious agent is
    A. infection
    B. immune reaction
    • C. inflammation
    D. phagocytosis
    E. detoxification

192. Inflammation is characterized by five distinct responses. These are
    A. redness, heat, swelling, hemorrhage, shock
    B. swelling, hemorrhage, hematoma, loss of function, pain
    C. heat, swelling, loss of function, paralysis
    • D. redness, heat, swelling, pain, altered function
    E. redness, swelling, pain, hemorrhage, shock

193. There are three types of healing: first, second, and third intention. Which of the following statements are true of first intention healing?
   - A. It is the most desirable
   - B. All levels of tissue heal at the same time
   - C. It usually leaves a wide, irregular scar
   - D. Healing of subcutaneous layer only
   - E. None of the above

194. What statements are true of second intention healing?
   - A. Healing is delayed because of infection
   - B. There is uneven union of tissues
   - C. Incisional hernia may occur
   - D. Healing is by granulation
   - E. All of the above

195. Third intention healing
   - A. follows gross infection
   - B. is extremely rare
   - C. is characterized by debridement
   - D. is common following bowel resections
   - E. none of the above

196. The healing process is also characterized by various time periods. The lag phase is when tissues are held together by fibrin and serum. What is the time period for the lag phase?
   - A. 4-7 days
   - B. 1-2 days
   - C. 7-10 days
   - D. 14 days
   - E. More than 21 days

197. The healing phase occurs when the wound edges are held together by connective tissue. This occurs around
   - A. 4-7 days
   - B. 7-14 days
   - C. 14-21 days
   - D. more than 21 days
   - E. none of the above

5. INFECTION

DIRECTIONS: Each of the questions or incomplete statements below is followed by five suggested answers or completions. Select the most appropriate answer(s).

A. Process of Infection

198. Immunity may be defined as
    A. unsusceptibility to a specific disease
    B. a naturally acquired trait
    C. an artificially acquired status
    • D. all of the above
    E. none of the above

199. Sepsis is
    A. a state of being free from infection
    • B. the presence of pathogenic organisms in the blood or tissues
    C. used to denote the presence of microorganisms known as opportunists
    D. the desired condition of a surgical wound
    E. A and D

200. Pathogenic microorganisms may enter the patient's body
    • A. from the patient's own skin during surgery
    • B. from contaminated surgical supplies
    • C. by droplets from respiratory tracts of the surgical team, and hair from surgical team
    D. from poor aseptic practices
    E. all of the above

201. Infection is
   A. white or yellow creamy material collected in the tissues
   B. morbid tissue reaction to disease, producing degeneration of tissues
   C. the entrance into the body tissues of pathogenic organisms
   D. the ability of microorganisms to cause disease
   E. none of the above

202. Natural immunity is
   - A. inborn, independent of previous experience
   B. gained in response to a foreign agent
   C. received through a vaccine
   D. received through a toxoid
   E. none of the above

203. Passive immunity is
   - A. after an infection with a known organism, doses of a specific antitoxin (antibodies) are given to combat toxins
   B. when a vaccine is administered
   C. when a toxoid is administered
   D. the production of neutralizing antibodies
   E. a nonentity

204. How might the patient be contaminated by the surgical team and/or operating room (OR)?
   - A. Moisture droplets from respiratory tract, open windows
   - B. Excessive handling of sterile supplies
   C. Proper time exposure in sterilization
   - D. Improper decontamination techniques of surgical environment and instrumentation
   E. All of the above

B. Prevention and Control of Infection

205. What is a bactericide?
   A. A freshly contaminated object
   - B. An agent which destroys bacteria
   C. An agent which inhibits the growth of bacteria
   D. A bacterial vaccine
   E. Viable bacteria in the circulating blood

206. If a wound is suppurating, it is
- A. said to be pus producing
- B. surgically clean
- C. superior healing potential
- D. the desired state of a new surgical wound
- E. the dwelling of Clostridium perfringens

207. What does it mean to terminally sterilize supplies?
- A. To make as clean as possible
- B. To sterilize articles after they have been used and before putting them into circulation again
- C. To remove pathogenic organisms but may not remove spore-forming organisms
- D. To soak in a chemical disinfectant for 5 min
- E. None of the above

208. If a surgical procedure is said to be septic, what does this mean?
- A. There is pathogenic bacteria and pus present and a certain procedure should be followed in order to contain the bacteria and destroy them without infecting personnel and supplies
- B. It is another way of saying that strict aseptic technique has been followed during a procedure
- C. At some time during the surgical procedure there has been a break in technique
- D. It applies to a procedure when an abscess is drained
- E. None of the above

209. Because we know bacteria do not fly but must be transported by vectors, how can bacteria be controlled in the air in the OR?
- A. Use of vacuum to clean floor
- B. Aeration of rooms overnight; windows should be closed an hour before the first case
- C. Daily damp-dusting of all surfaces
- D. Proper cleaning of air ventilation systems
- E. All of the above

210. Other methods of controlling the cleanliness of the OR are
- A. control of traffic within the suite
- B. proper attire worn by everyone in the department
- C. constant vigilance in cleaning of floors, walls, furniture, ceiling, and ventilators and care of trash
- D. daily spraying with a disinfectant
- E. hosing down the OR each day

211. A simple but great contribution to infection control advocated by Semmelweis was the
   A. use of sterilization for instrumentation
   •B. washing of hands between patient contacts
   C. use of antibiotics
   D. none of the above
   E. all of the above

212. What great man marked the beginning of the antiseptic area and the modern age of surgery?
   A. Black
   B. Pasteur
   • C. Lister
   D. Pore
   E. None of the above

213. Proper OR attire should consist of
   A. clean OR apparel
   B. shoe covers
   C. mask
   D. surgical hat or hood
   - E. all of the above

214. An object or substance is considered sterile when it is
   A. clean
   • B. free of all living microorganisms
   • C. incapable of producing any form of life
   D. all of the above
   E. none of the above

215. Which of the following are no longer acceptable for use in OR because they have a very low filtration efficiency?
   A. Cloth caps
   • B. Cloth/gauze masks
   C. Paper gowns
   D. All of the above
   E. None of the above

216. Proper adherence to aseptic techniques eliminates or minimizes modes and sources of contamination. Examples of this would be
   A. top surface to 3 in. below of a dried table is considered sterile
   •B. a sterile package once opened is considered unsterile
   •C. the edge of a bottle cap is considered contaminated once the cap has been removed from the bottle
   D. all of the above
   E. none of the above

217. When pouring solution into a sterile receptacle
   • A. the circulating nurse maintains a safe margin to avoid contamination
   • B. the circulating nurse should pour solution without reaching over sterile field
   • C. the scrub nurse should hold receptacle away from sterile field
   D. none of the above
   E. all of the above

218. Clean shoe covers should be worn when returning to the restricted areas of the OR to
   A. maintain cleanliness of shoes
   • B. prevent cross-contamination from other areas
   C. allow for maximum bacterial protection
   D. to prevent skidding on slippery floors
   E. none of the above

219. Synthetic disposable masks must have a filtration efficiency of
   A. 85% or more
   B. 90% or more
   • C. 95% or more
   D. 100%
   E. none of the above

220. Which of the following should never be worn within restricted areas of the surgical suite?
   • A. Jewelry
   • B. Street clothes
   • C. Silk slips
   • D. False eyelashes
   E. None of the above

6. STERILIZATION AND DISINFECTION

DIRECTIONS: Each of the questions or incomplete statements below is followed by five suggested answers or completions. Select the most appropriate answer(s).

---

221. An antiseptic is an agent
    A. which prevents or eliminates microorganisms from animate objects
    B. which prevents or eliminates microorganisms from inanimate objects
    C. which is capable of killing spore-forming organisms
    D. such as Lysol
    E. such as Cidex

222. A disinfectant is an agent
    A. which prevents or eliminates microorganisms from animate objects
    B. which destroys microorganisms on inanimate objects
    C. capable of killing spore-forming organisms
    D. such as Lysol
    E. none of the above

223. A bacteriostatic agent is an agent
    A. capable of destroying spores
    B. which destroys microorganisms
    C. which inhibits the growth of microorganisms but does not necessarily destroy them
    D. used only on animate objects
    E. used only on inanimate objects

224. What is a spore?
   • A. It is a protective device of certain bacteria
   B. It is a classification of bacteria
   C. It is an agent which is used to destroy certain bacteria when the usual methods have not done so
   D. It is a bacterial cell which does not normally invade tissue
   E. It is the causative agent of a septic case

225. What is sanitation?
   A. The process by which all used articles in the OR are rendered free from pathogenic organisms
   B. A method of killing spore-forming organisms
   • C. A process of cleaning with soap and water and reducing the number of organisms to safe levels according to public health standards
   D. A method of inhibiting the growth of bacteria
   E. All of the above

226. What is sterilization?
   • A. Removing or killing <u>all</u> microbes
   B. Removing or killing pathogenic organisms
   C. Removing aerobic organisms
   D. Killing aerobic and anaerobic organisms
   E. Removing and killing spores

227. What is it necessary to know about the material being sterilized?
   A. The type of material it is, e.g., metal, rubber
   B. Whether it is grossly contaminated or minimally contaminated
   C. Whether it is smooth, irregular, hinged
   • D. A and C
   E. None of the above

228. One of the most common methods of sterilizing supplies for surgery is steam under pressure. Bacterial cell destruction in the autoclave is caused by
   • A. heat—it coagulates the protein in the cell
   B. the replacement of steam for air
   C. the physical cleansing and then exposure to steam
   D. 47 lb of pressure, which is the usual amount found in the hospital autoclave
   E. the excessive amount of moisture present in the autoclave in the form of steam

229. The chamber gauge of the autoclave reads 27-30 lb/sq in. What is the temperature reading?
   A. 250° F
   •B. 270° F
   C. 290° F
   D. 240° F
   E. 200° F

230. The chamber gauge of the autoclave reads 17-20 lb/sq in. What is the temperature reading?
   •A. 250° F
   B. 270° F
   C. 290° F
   D. 240° F
   E. 200° F

231. What is the most resistant form of bacteria and what sterilizing agents must aim to destroy?
   A. Streptococcus aureus
   B. Staphylococcus albus
   C. Staphylococcal toxins
   •D. Bacterial spores
   E. Hemolytic streptococci

232. Once a load has been placed in the autoclave, what should be checked to ascertain whether the autoclave is functioning correctly?
   A. The gauge which records the pressure in the jacket
   B. The gauge which records the pressure in the chamber
   C. The gauge which records the temperature
   D. The graphic chart which indicates temperature and time exposure
   •E. All of the above

233. The usual exposure time for wrapped supplies is
   •A. 30 min at 250° F
   B. 30 min at 270° F
   C. 15 min at 250° F
   •D. 15 min at 270° F
   E. 15 min at 300° F

234. The usual exposure for unwrapped instruments is
   A. 10 min at 250° F
   B. 15 min at 270° F
   C. 7 min at 270° F
   •D. 3 min at 270° F
   E. 5 min at 300° F

235. Which of the following is a disadvantage of the instrument-washer-sterilizer? It
   - A. has a long cycle, usually 20 min
   - B. is expensive to use
   - C. corrodes glassware
   - D. is difficult to maintain in working condition
   - E. sterilizes instruments only when on for 7 min at 270° F

236. In a high-vacuum sterilizer
   - A. exposure time is 3-10 min at 270 °F
   - B. exposure time is usually over 10 min at 275° F
   - C. positive destruction of bacteria must be checked with every load which is run
   - D. a temperature of over 300° F is reached
   - E. all air is kept within the chamber

237. When something is gas sterilized, what is the name of the gas that is used?
   - A. Nitrous oxide
   - B. Ethylene oxide
   - C. Ethylene chloride
   - D. Fluothane
   - E. Carbon dioxide

238. When ethylene oxide gas is used to sterilize articles, what other gases are used in conjunction with it to decrease flammability and explosiveness?
   - A. Carbon dioxide
   - B. Cyclopropane
   - C. Carbon monoxide
   - D. Oxygen
   - E. Freon

239. All material for ethylene oxide sterilization must
   - A. be thoroughly cleaned
   - B. be prepared and held in an area where humidity is 30% or more
   - C. have plugs and stylets removed so gas can penetrate freely
   - D. contain a biological monitor to assure positive assurance that sterilization conditions were achieved
   - E. all of the above

240. Ethylene oxide is
   A. relatively inexpensive
   B. expensive
   C. highly flammable
   D. all of the above
   E. B and C

241. Aeration of ethylene oxide sterilized items
   A. is absolutely necessary
   B. is done only if there is adequate time
   C. may be carried out in a clean, well-ventilated storage area
   D. may be carried out in the aeration chamber
   E. must be carried out in a high-oxygen and high-humidity area

242. Another method of sterilizing supplies is electron beam sterilization. This is mainly used
   A. in the OR
   B. in cardiopulmonary labs
   C. in central supply
   D. in surgical supply manufacturing plants
   E. for anesthesia equipment

243. What are some factors concerning time which should be remembered when using a disinfectant?
   A. The object being disinfected (flat, irregular)
   B. The nature of the organisms
   C. The limitations of the disinfectant
   D. The temperature of the room
   E. All of the above

244. Which of the following is true of mercurials?
   A. Extremely potent; bacteriostatic
   B. Sporicidal
   C. Poor germicides; bacteriostatic agents only
   D. Effective against vegetative bacteria only
   E. Should be used only on furniture

245. An example of a phenolic compound is
   A. Zephiran
   B. Cidex
   C. Betadine
   D. Lysol
   E. Metaphen

246. Phenolic compounds are
- A. good germicides for furniture
- B. good antiseptics
- C. able to kill spores
- D. able to kill viruses
- E. none of the above

247. Chlorine compounds are
- A. good disinfectants for floors, bedpans, urinals
- B. corrosive to metal instruments
- C. corrosive to articles made of rubber
- D. harmless as a germicidal
- E. none of the above

248. An example of a quaternary ammonium compound is
- A. Thorexin
- B. Zephiran
- C. Betadine
- D. Cidex
- E. Lysol

249. Tincture of iodine
- A. is an excellent skin antiseptic
- B. is irritating to tissues
- C. stains
- D. kills viruses, fungi, bacteria
- E. all of the above

250. Formaldehyde solution is
- A. irritating to tissue
- B. sporicidal
- C. a nonirritating solution when mixed with alcohol
- D. nonirritating solution when mixed with water
- E. none of the above

251. An example of glutaraldehyde is
- A. Thesiodyne
- B. Zephiran
- C. Cidex
- D. hexachlorophene
- E. Lysol

252. When a disinfectant has been used, what are some precautions to follow?
   A. Article must be used as soon as it is removed from the disinfectant solution
   B. Important to realize that there are no limitations to any disinfectants which are on the market today
   C. Article should be rinsed thoroughly with sterile water before it is used
   D. Article should be rinsed thoroughly with tap water before it is used
   E. When soaking an article such as a laparoscope, be sure that no disinfectant solution is allowed into the lumen of the scope

253. If articles that have been sterilized are wet at the end of the cycle, many things could be the causative agent. These might be
   A. improper packing and loading of sterilizer
   B. malfunctioning of autoclave
   C. placing all types of packages on side
   D. leaving all wrapped articles in autoclave for hours
   E. none of the above

254. All supplies which are wrapped and sterilized in the hospital are marked with an expiration date. What does this indicate?
   A. One month after the date which appears on the package or tag, the article must be reprocessed
   B. The package may be used up to 6 months after the date which appears
   C. The package must not be used after the date which appears
   D. The package may be used after the date which appears, but a report is usually required
   E. None of the above

255. Which of the following is a quality of a proper packaging material?
   A. It must be penetrable to steam and/or ethylene oxide sterilants
   B. It must permit easy removal of the product for aseptic presentation
   C. It must be a triple thickness
   D. It must be expensive
   E. It must be reliable barrier to microorganisms but not dust particles

256. Muslin wrappers
- A. are the least expensive of packaging materials
- B. are expensive, but economical once initial investment is made
- C. are rated high in mechanical strength
- D. need to be inspected for worn spots, tears, and holes
- E. are no longer used in most hospitals and have been replaced by polyethylene pouches

257. Nonwoven wrap or textile is a one-time/one-use product which is found as the wrapper of disposable goods or as disposable drapes. Regarding nonwoven wrap
- A. it is strong, water repellent, flexible, and easy to use
- B. steam sterilization and gas sterilization do not change quality of item
- C. shelf-life is better or more reliable than muslin-wrapped goods
- D. it is strong but difficult to use and susceptible to contamination by water
- E. none of the above

258. Shelf-life periods generally accepted in most hospitals are
- A. paper and muslin goods: 21-30 days; with dust covers, 6 months-1 year
- B. paper and muslin goods: 30-90 days; with dust covers, indefinite time
- C. heat-sealed or hermetically sealed items: 6 months-1 year
- D. prepackaged sterile items: until damaged or opened
- E. tape-sealed, plastic-packaged items: 3-4 months

259. When sterilizing muslin or linen items, what is important?
- A. All linen must be inspected for holes
- B. Large linen items should be fan-folded to allow adequate steam penetration
- C. Items should be sterilized for 30 min at 250° F
- D. Metalware should be included in pack
- E. All of the above

260. Electrical equipment such as bone saws or drills may be sterilized by
   A. ethylene oxide
   B. steam under pressure
   C. Cidex
   D. dry heat
   E. none of the above

261. Vaseline or mineral oil may be sterilized by
   A. ethylene oxide
   B. steam under pressure
   C. Cidex
   D. radiation
   E. dry heat

262. If a tray or instruments is wrapped, it is sterilized for
   A. 0 min at 250° F
   B. 3 min at 270° F
   C. 30 min at 250° F
   D. 20 min at 350° F
   E. 60 min at 400° F

263. When preparing rubber goods for sterilization by ethylene oxide, it is imperative that products
   A. be conductive
   B. are moistened
   C. are completely dry
   D. be of high-quality material
   E. none of the above

III

CARE OF THE PATIENT

7. THE SURGICAL PATIENT

DIRECTIONS: Each of the questions or incomplete statements below is followed by five suggested answers or completions. Select the most appropriate answer(s).

---

264. The purpose of care during the preoperative period is to
    A. prepare the patient physically to withstand the effects of surgery
    B. prepare the patient and the OR staff for the proposed surgery
    C. prepare the patient, both physically and psychologically, to withstand the effects of anesthesia and surgery
    D. be sure the patient understands in detail all aspects of the surgical procedure
    E. medicate the patient

265. Patients express their anxiety by
    A. open expression of fears
    B. indifference
    C. hostility
    D. all of the above
    E. none of the above

266. Patients are premedicated to produce a desirable physical state. Reactions to drugs can be noted by
    A. excessive talking by patient
    B. profuse perspiration
    C. drowsiness
    D. complaints of dizziness
    E. complaints of headache

267. When transporting patients from units to the OR
- A. proceed to patient's room, tell him who you are, and put him on the stretcher
- B. go to ward, check with person at desk, pick up patient's complete chart, proceed to patient's room
- C. ask patient his name
- D. introduce yourself and check patient's wrist band for identification
- E. help patient move onto stretcher, being sure locks are on stretcher and you have enough help to move patient

268. When transporting patients who are on precautions because of a communicable disease, you would
- A. be sure the patient puts on a clean gown
- B. use a clean cotton blanket to cover the patient
- C. have the patient wear a high-efficiency disposable mask
- D. wear a gown and mask
- E. all of the above

269. Preoperative shaving of the patient in the OR should be avoided because of which of the following reasons?
- A. Prolonged anesthesia time
- B. Loose hair from skin preparation may enter wound
- C. Encroachment of OR time
- D. All of the above
- E. A and B only

270. The skin is the body's first line of defense against disease. A break in the skin
- A. may allow microorganisms to enter the body
- B. if it is small, is insignificant and no danger
- C. should be reported to the OR charge nurse
- D. can be cleansed and dressed with no aftereffects
- E. all of the above

271. The position which is used for the patient is decided by the
- A. surgeon
- B. anesthesiologist
- C. circulating nurse
- D. surgeon and anesthesiologist
- E. all of the above

272. Dorsal or supine position is when the patient lies flat on his back. When using this position, one must be sure that
   A. the head is in line with the body and that the arms are straight and secured alongside the body with palms down (unless one arm is out on a board for IV)
   B. a large pillow is placed under the midback
   C. a knee strap is secured tightly, directly over the knees
   D. the heels and feet are protected and supported with padding
   E. the body skin surfaces are not in contact with one another

273. A modification of the dorsal or supine position is the Trendelenburg. This position is
   A. used for gall bladder surgery
   B. when the patient's head is lowered
   C. used for operation on the organs of the pelvic cavity
   D. used to overcome shock
   E. where the head of the patient is lowered and the lower portion of the table is dropped slightly (being sure patient's knees are over the breaking point of the lower part of the table)

274. When reverse Trendelenburg is used
   A. the abdominal viscera tend to fall toward the lower part of abdominal cavity
   B. the patient's circulation improves
   C. extra support such as foot board and body straps must be used
   D. the patient is in a normally comfortable position
   E. none of the above

275. Regarding modified Fowler's position
   A. it is a semi-upright position, backrest elevated 45°, knees flexed over break, footboard supports feet
   B. hands and arms need to be supported
   C. it is used for some neurological, ENT procedures
   D. it is used for perineal procedures
   E. all of the above

276. Lithotomy position is a variation of dorsal position. Some precautionary measures are
   A. patient's buttocks should be positioned and maintained at lower break of table to prevent lumbosacral strain
   B. stirrups must be level
   C. legs are positioned in stirrups simultaneously and removed simultaneously. Unilateral movement can affect hemodynamics
   D. position arms loosely over abdomen
   E. all of the above

277. Lateral position is
   A. used for chest surgery
   B. placement of the patient on his or her side
   C. one that requires much support, such as straps and padding
   D. used for kidney surgery
   E. all of the above

278. When kidney surgery is done
   A. patient is placed in dorsal position
   B. patient is placed on side with area between iliac crest and costal margin directly over break in table between back and seat
   C. only bottom half of table is lowered
   D. table is flexed using slight reverse Trendelenberg position
   E. it is preferable to use a kidney bar attachment

279. Prone position is when the patient lies on abdomen, face down. This position
   A. is used for rectal, back, and spine operations but carries hazards because of intra-abdominal pressure interfering with action of the diaphragm
   B. can be adapted into jackknife or Kraske position
   C. requires special attention to head and eyes
   D. requires that the patient's weight must not rest on elbows and that a support be placed under the ankles
   E. all of the above

8. ANESTHESIA

DIRECTIONS: Each of the questions or incomplete statements below is followed by five suggested answers or completions. Select the most appropriate answer(s).

---

280. Anesthesia
    A. is a state of unconsciousness
    • B. is the absence of essentially all sensation
    • C. renders the patient in such a state that the operation can be carried out without discomfort
    D. should not in any way disturb the normal physiology of the body
    • E. produces optimal conditions for speedy performance of surgery

281. General anesthesia is when the agent permeates the entire body and affects all its functions. The agents are transported by the bloodstream, which absorbs them
    A. from the respiratory system when agents are given by inhalation
    B. directly, when agents are given by IV
    C. from mucosa when agents are administered into an organ such as the rectum
    • D. all of the above
    E. none of the above

282. What are the stages of general anesthesia?
    • A. Induction, excitement, operative, overdose
    B. Induction, operative
    C. Induction, excitement, operative
    D. Induction, excitement
    E. None of the above

283. Regarding regional anesthesia
- A. there is injection or application of the drug along the course of a nerve
- B. an example of an agent is Xylocaine
- C. the patient immediately falls asleep when agent is administered
- D. the patient experiences pain during procedure
- E. the patient remains awake and does not experience pain during operative procedure

284. When a nerve block is done
- A. the agent is injected directly into tissues
- B. procaine or Xylocaine may be used
- C. the agent is injected just outside the dura
- D. the agent is injected in and around the main nerve trunk at a site between the operative site and entry of the nerve into the spinal cord to cause blockage of painful stimuli
- E. it is only for dental surgery

285. Which of the following statements are true concerning spinal anesthesia?
- A. Anesthetic agent injected into the subarachnoid space and acts on the nerves as they emerge from the spinal cord
- B. It is used for surgery above the diaphragm
- C. Anesthetic agent injected into the dura and acts on the nerves as they emerge from the spinal cord
- D. It is used for surgery on the lower limbs, perineum, sometimes the gall bladder
- E. It provides good relaxation of muscles

286. Cardiac arrest is a serious complication and an emergency situation in the OR, but it can happen anywhere. Which of the following steps should be taken when cardiac arrest occurs?
- A. Observe for absence of respiration, pulse, and dilation of pupils
- B. Quickly follow ABC (airway, breathing, circulation)
- C. Open airway by hyperextension of the head
- D. Give artificial breathing at a mouth-to-mouth rate of 12/min, apply artificial respiration by closed chest massage at a rate of 60/min
- E. All of the above

287. In the OR, which of the following emergency equipment should be available for treatment of patients in cardiac arrest?
- A. Suction, airways, oxygen, anesthesia machine
- B. Cardiac monitor, pacer, defibrillator
- C. Special stimulant drugs, syringes, needles, tracheostomy set
- D. All of the above
- E. None of the above

288. These hazards can be controlled by
- A. keeping humidity below 55%
- B. installing explosion-proof switches, motors, etc.
- C. each member of staff putting a nail in the heel of his shoe for grounding
- D. use of conductive flooring, and casters on furniture and all other items in contact with floor
- E. proper clothing worn by personnel and patient, avoiding wools, rayons, and synthetics

289. What can be done to reduce the health hazards that exist for OR personnel because of anesthetic gas waste?
- A. General anesthetics must be kept to a minimum
- B. Some type of gas waste disposal or evacuation system should be installed in the OR suite
- C. Installation of an atmospheric monitoring program
- D. Use of only spinal anesthesia
- E. Use of only locals or nerve blocks

IV

OPERATING ROOM TECHNIQUES

9. GENERAL PRINCIPLES

DIRECTIONS: Each of the questions or incomplete statements below is followed by five suggested answers or completions. Select the most appropriate answer(s).

---

290. A successful operation must be an infection-free process. This is accomplished by
    A. eliminating bacterial contamination as much as possible
    B. development of a "sterile" conscience in all OR personnel
    C. installing ultraviolet lights in each OR
    D. being sure the patient is free of bacterial contamination
    E. none of the above

291. The rules of asepsis involve four simple points. Which of the following is NOT one of the four points?
    A. Know what is sterile
    B. Know what is not sterile
    C. Keep the two apart
    D. Remedy contamination immediately
    E. All of the above

292. Surgical drapes should be
    A. fluid resistant
    B. correct size for adequate draping
    C. made of wicking material
    D. shaken well to remove wrinkles
    E. positioned accurately

293. The advantages of plastic incisional drapes are that they
   A. can be fitted to irregular body surfaces
   B. wall off contaminated areas
   C. form a complete seal, as they are impermeable
   D. allow good visibility of anatomical landmarks
   E. all of the above

294. The epidermis is the outer layer of skin.
   A. It is where resident bacteria are found
   B. It contains the hair roots and sweat glands
   C. It contains the nerves and blood vessels
   D. It contains the transient bacteria
   E. It varies in thickness

295. The subungual area is
   A. the deep layer of skin
   B. where the resident bacteria are formed
   C. where infected hangnails develop
   D. under the fingernail and very difficult to clean
   E. an especially contaminated area

296. If a time method of scrubbing is used, the usual time is
   A. 5 min
   B. 3 min
   C. 7-10 min
   D. 10-12 min
   E. none of the above

297. After drying the hands and arms, the gown is donned by handling under aseptic conditions in which of the following ways?
   A. The gown is handled on the inner side close to the neckband
   B. The gown is held high above the head before opening
   C. The gown is unfolded so that the inner surface faces the wearer
   D. The arms are placed in armholes; then the gown can be pulled on by grasping the surface directly above the elbow
   E. Put arms into armholes and have circulator pull gown on by grasping inner surface of back

298. To properly remove the gown after surgery
- • A. circulator should untie gown
- B. scrubbed person unties gown
- • C. grasp gown at shoulder seam
- • D. remove gown down over gloved hands
- E. be sure gloves are removed first

299. The procedure for donning sterile gloves by the closed method is
- • A. to prevent bare hands from coming in contact with the outside of the glove
- • B. the hands are extended to the edge of the wristlets of the gown
- C. the hands are pushed through the cuff as the gloves are pulled in place
- • D. to adjust each glove properly once both hands are gloved
- E. to wipe excessive powder from gloves

300. A gowned and gloved scrub person assists another gowned individual using which of the following techniques?
- • A. Gloved person places fingers of each hand beneath everted cuff
- B. Palm of glove is always facing you
- • C. The cuff is stretched to open the glove
- D. All of the above
- E. None of the above

301. Reusable cotton cloth drapes should have a thread count of
- A. 140-160/sq in.
- • B. 288/sq in.
- C. 480/sq in.
- D. 320/sq in.
- E. none of the above

302. Advantages of disposable drapes are that they
- A. are lightweight
- B. reduce the hazards of contamination
- C. are flame and moisture resistant
- D. are lint free
- ✓ E. all of the above

303. There are a variety of standard drapes that allow for economy of time and body motion. Examples would be
   - A. whole or plain sheet
   - B. slit sheets
   - C. laparotomy sheet
   - D. perineal sheet
   - E. all of the above

304. Drapes should NOT be
   - A. shaken
   - B. flipped
   - C. perforated by towel clips
   - D. used if sterility is questionable
   - E. all of the above

305. Between surgical procedures, personnel should
   - A. remove gowns
   - B. remove gloves
   - C. place both disposable and reusable items in proper receptacles
   - D. place wet linen in the center of the laundry bundle to prevent soaking through
   - E. all of the above

306. The preoperative assessment of the patient is necessary to determine
   - A. psychological preparation of the patient
   - B. physical preparation of the patient
   - C. past medical/surgical history
   - D. patient concerns related to surgery
   - E. all of the above

307. Routine tests performed prior to surgical intervention are
   - A. chest x-ray
   - B. ECG
   - C. urinalysis
   - D. CBC
   - E. all of the above

308. When the patient arrives in the surgical suite, the first item addressed is the
   - A. patency of IV site
   - B. preoperative shave
   - C. patient's name band
   - D. patient's chart and completion of the preoperative testing
   - E. none of the above

309. The most commonly ordered pre-anesthetic medications are
   A. barbiturates
   B. narcotics
   C. anticholinergics
   D. tranquilizers
   E. none of the above

310. Temperature in the OR should be controlled at
   A. 68-75° F
   B. 68-72° F
   C. 65-70° F
   D. 72-75° F
   E. none of the above

311. Humidity in the OR should be controlled at a minimum of
   A. 40%
   B. 45%
   C. 50%
   D. 55%
   E. none of the above

312. When using an electrosurgical unit, the connection from the patient to the machine should be checked if the surgeon continually requests high settings. Which of the following should be noted?
   A. Patient-plate contact
   B. Placement of plate in relation to operative site
   C. Inadequate connection of cable to plate
   D. Inadequate connection of plate/cable at the unit
   E. All of the above

313. A standard procedure for care and use of electrosurgical equipment should include which of the following?
   A. Kinks and curls in cord
   B. Cord breakage
   C. Two-prong plug for safety
   D. Personnel qualifications for use of equipment
   E. Check before each use

A. Duties of the Technician Assisting in Circulating Duties

314. The circulating technician assists the circulating nurse. In order to do this, he must understand
   A. sterilization and disinfection
   B. position
   C. aseptic technique
   D. use of special equipment
   E. all of the above

315. Accessory parts to the OR table would include
   A. anesthesia screen
   B. cassette holder
   C. wristlets
   D. stirrups
   E. all of the above

316. The duties of the circulator are to care for the patient, care for all needs of the team, care for all records, and maintain the proper environment. Other important duties of the RN only are
   A. care of the specimens
   B. sponge count
   C. preparing the dressing
   D. weighing sponges, estimating blood loss
   E. all medications

317. At the finish of a case, the circulator
   A. secures the dressing and connects all drainage tubes properly
   B. leaves the room until the time arrives for the next case
   C. obtains help and properly moves the patient off the table and onto a stretcher or bed
   D. takes specimens and records out of the room to designated areas
   E. leaves the patient for the anesthesiologist and orderly to transport to ward or recovery area

318. In the care of the OR after a case
- A. the cleaning should be thorough and efficient with an effective germicide
- B. a different technique is used after an infected case
- C. there is no such thing as a "septic case"
- D. a mop and solution is the most dependable method for cleaning floors
- E. none of the above

319. The most effective way of cleaning the OR floor is
- A. spraying with detergent
- B. mopping with hot water
- C. mopping with detergent
- D. wet vacuuming
- E. dry vacuuming

10. SUTURE MATERIAL

DIRECTIONS: Each of the questions or incomplete statements below is followed by five suggested answers or completions. Select the most appropriate answer(s).

---

320. Suture material may be absorbable or nonabsorbable. An example of absorbable suture material is
   •A. chromic gut
   B. polyester
   •C. ribbon gut
   •D. plain catgut
   E. synthetic with teflon

321. Regarding cotton, nylon, and linen (which are non-absorbable sutures)
   A. all are used commonly for ligatures
   •B. all can be used for internal suturing
   •C. only cotton and nylon are commonly used
   D. none are used for ligatures
   E. all are used only for skin stitches

322. Stainless steel is an iron ore alloy which
   • A. is used for internal and external suturing
   B. is produced only in monofilament strands
   • C. ranges in size from 7 to 6-0
   . D. is sometimes classified in sizes 18-40
   E. can be used in orthopedic surgery to secure vitalium prosthetic appliances

323. Suture material wedged into a needle of the same diameter is called
   A. suture ligature
   • B. atraumatic
   C. through and through
   D. ligature
   E. none of the above

324. An interrupted suture is short and used for only one stitch, which is tied and cut. A continuous suture is long and many stitches can be taken before tying and cutting. Through-and-through sutures are
•A. called tension, retention, or stay sutures
•B. usually heavy, nonabsorbable material
C. routinely used on all abdominal surgery
•D. placed a distance from the incision
E. used to close the skin layer

325. An example of polypropylene suture is
A. nylon
•B. proline
•C. surgilene
D. catgut
E. none of the above

326. An example of a synthetic polyamide material is
•A. Dermalon
•B. Surgilon
•C. Nurolon
D. Dacron
E. all of the above

327. Which of the following is a strand of suture material threaded or swaged on a needle?
A. Ligature
B. Buried suture
•C. Suture ligature
D. Interrupted
E. None of the above

328. A strand of suture material used to tie off blood vessels is known as
A. suture
B. purse string
•C. ligature
D. absorbable
E. none of the above

329. An autosuture instrument used to ligate and divide omental vessels is the
A. EEA
B. GIA
•C. LDS
D. TA-90
E. TA-55

11. SPONGES/NEEDLES/DRAINS

DIRECTIONS: Each of the questions or incomplete statements below is followed by a list of suggested answers or completions. Select the most appropriate answer(s).

---

330. A suture needle is made of tempered steel and
    - A. has a distinctive shape
    - B. is strong enough to pass through tissue
    - C. is made so that the eye is easy to thread
    - D. is the proper size to carry a suture but cause no trauma
    - E. all of the above

331. Parts of the needle are the
    - A. handling portion
    - B. eye
    - C. shaft
    - D. holder
    - E. point

332. Sponges used in the operative field must be
    - A. x-ray detectable
    - B. used economically
    - C. counted carefully
    - D. nontraumatic
    - E. all of the above

333. The sponge count
    - A. should be recorded by a registered professional nurse
    - B. is an act carrying legal responsibility
    - C. is a routine set up by the Joint Commission on Hospital Accreditation
    - D. is a routine set by each individual hospital
    - E. is usually done only if the surgeon desires or requests it

334. Drains are used to remove fluid or air from body cavities and tissue. They are usually placed
A. in all abdominal wounds
B. where oozing of blood may occur
C. in the chest cavity to remove air
D. so as to drain dependently
E. in all infected wounds

335. Catheters are a type of drain most commonly used on the urinary system. They are of many types, such as the
A. Foley
B. Penrose
C. Malecot
D. Pezzer
E. all of the above

336. A Levine tube is used to drain the stomach. A type of sump drain is usually used in
A. appendectomy wounds
B. areas with large amounts of drainage
C. all chest wounds
D. the gall bladder and ducts
E. none of the above

337. A tube inserted for enteral feeding is a
A. catheter
B. gastrostomy tube
C. Levine tube
D. Malecot
E. Pezzer

338. Which of the following is a portable, self-contained drainage system?
A. Penrose
B. Hemovac
C. Pleurovac system
D. All of the above
E. None of the above

339. Advantages of having no dressing are which of the following?
A. Allows for observation of the incisional site
B. Prevents possible adhesive tape burns
C. Increases maneuverability for patient
D. Minimizes adverse response to operation by patients
E. All of the above

340. Which of the following may be used when frequent dressing changes are anticipated?
A. Operative site transparent dressing
• B. Montgomery straps
C. Abdominal binder
D. Ace bandages
E. None of the above

341. When threading a surgical needle, the scrub nurse should pull how many inches through the eye of the needle?
A. 1
B. 2
C. 3
• D. 4
E. None of the above

342. If a drainage tube is inserted in the wound, the tube may be anchored to the skin with which of the following sutures?
A. Absorbable
• B. Nonabsorbable
C. Nylon
D. Cotton
E. Silk

12. INSTRUMENTATION

DIRECTIONS: Each of the questions or incomplete statements below is followed by a list of suggested answers or completions. Select the most appropriate answer(s).

---

343. Instruments are classified as
 •A. cutting, clamping
 B. exploring, suction
 • C. grasping, exposing
 D. dissecting
 E. all of the above

344. Metzenbaum scissors are common instruments found in many surgical set-ups. These scissors are usually used for
 A. suture scissors
 • B. gentle, fine dissection
 C. moderately heavy dissection
 D. heavy dissection
 E. all plastic surgery

345. Bandage scissors would be used on a surgical procedure such as
 A. hysterectomy
 B. uterine suspension
 • C. cesarean section
 D. vaginal repair
 E. laparotomy

346. Mixter clamps are often referred to as
 A. graspers
 B. hemostats
 • C. right-angle clamps
 D. tissue forceps
 E. none of the above

347. Lahey clamps are most commonly used for
   - A. gentle tissue grasping
   - B. intestinal procedures
   - C. heavy tissue and specimen grasping
   - D. peritoneal grasping
   - E. closure procedures

348. Babcock clamps are usually found in the instrument kit for
   - A. breast surgery
   - B. intestinal surgery
   - C. amputations
   - D. gastric surgery
   - E. all of the above

349. Payr clamps are for use in
   - A. intestinal surgery
   - B. rectal surgery
   - C. gastric surgery
   - D. gall bladder surgery
   - E. bladder surgery

350. Witlaner retractors are most commonly used in
   - A. surgery on the back
   - B. surgery on the extremities
   - C. some vascular surgery
   - D. surgery of the thyroid gland
   - E. surgery of the thoracic cavity

351. An Auvard weighted speculum would be used on
   - A. bladder surgery
   - B. vaginal or cervical procedures
   - C. rectal surgery
   - D. urethral surgery
   - E. none of the above

352. A Graves speculum is used for procedures on the
   - A. nose
   - B. urethra
   - C. vagina
   - D. ear
   - E. cervix

353. A Satinsky clamp is usually found in the instrument set-up for
- A. lung surgery
- • B. cardiovascular surgery
- C. gastric surgery
- D. intestinal surgery
- E. none of the above

354. Hank dilators are used in surgery on the
- A. common bile ducts
- B. esophagus
- C. rectum
- • D. uterine cervix
- E. all of the above

355. Vulsellum tenaculi are commonly found in the set-up for surgery on the
- A. muscles of the extremities
- • B. uterus
- C. thyroid
- D. anus
- E. all of the above

356. Bulldog clamps are
- A. skin clamps
- B. large muscle clamps
- • C. small vascular clamps
- • D. very often counted during a procedure
- E. none of the above

357. An Alexander is
- A. a retractor
- B. a vascular clamp
- • C. a rib raspatory
- D. found in most orthopedic kits
- • E. found in most thoracic kits

358. A Gaylor biopsy forcep is usually used on the
- A. bronchus
- B. liver
- C. esophagus
- D. sigmoid
- • E. cervix

359. Yankauer is the name for a
   A. hemostat
   B. needle holder
   • C. suction tip
   D. retractor
   E. none of the above

360. A Castroviejo caliper would be used in
   A. cardiovascular surgery
   B. neurosurgery
   C. ear surgery
   • D. eye surgery
   E. nose surgery

361. Gouges are usually used on
   A. neurosurgical procedures
   • B. orthopedic procedures
   C. cardiovascular procedures
   D. gastrointestinal procedures
   E. none of the above

362. A Doyen is
   A. a needle holder
   • B. a rib raspatory
   C. a nasal rongeur
   D. a commissurotomy knife
   E. an obstetrical forcep

363. Gigli saws are usually used in
   A. orthopedic surgery
   B. nasal surgery
   C. mastoid surgery
   • D. surgery on the skull
   E. none of the above

364. Bethune shears are used on the
   A. vertebrae
   B. leg
   • C. ribs
   D. skull
   E. all of the above

365. A Ferris-Smith knife is most commonly used for
• A. skin grafting
B. amputation
C. tonsil removal
D. nasal septum procedures
E. none of the above

366. Kerrison rongeurs are used most frequently in
A. orthopedic surgery
• B. neurosurgery
C. common duct
D. ENT surgery
E. all of the above

367. Mayo scoops are usually found in the set-up for surgery on the
• A. gall bladder
B. kidney
C. stomach
D. bladder
E. none of the above

368. Hill retractors most frequently are used on
A. gynecological surgery
B. urethral surgery
• C. rectal surgery
D. eye surgery
E. none of the above

369. A Jackson forceps is used for
A. catheter insertion
• B. foreign body removal
C. nasal dressing
D. uterine dressing
E. general use

370. Instruments should be checked for
A. evenly meshed serrations
B. smoothly gliding ratchets
C. evenly closed jaws
D. sharpness (scissors, chisels, etc.)
• E. all of the above

371. Ultrasonic cleaning is done by use of
   A. high-steam pressure
   B. electronic waves
   • C. high-frequency sound waves
   D. water under high pressure
   E. none of the above

372. To clean the lumen, suction, and light channels of endoscopes, what would be used?
   • A. Long, narrow brushes
   • B. Long pipe cleaners
   C. Steel wool
   D. Pledgets
   E. None of the above

373. Soiled instruments, sponges, etc., should not be handled with uncovered hands. The purpose of this recommendation is to
   A. prevent staining of the hand with blood
   • B. avoid contamination by organisms from the patient
   C. prevent contact with fat cells deposited on instruments and sponges
   D. all of the above
   E. none of the above

374. Which of the following is true of ligation clips?
   • A. May be used to ligate vessels, nerves, ducts
   B. Can be applied to the skin
   • C. Are available in varied sizes
   D. Are used for tissue approximation
   E. All of the above

375. Stapling instruments are used for
   A. application of fine stainless steel staples formed into a "B" shape
   B. resection
   C. transection
   D. creation of anastomoses
   • E. all of the above

376. OR nurses and technicians may be responsible for
A. final selection of the proper stapling cartridge
B. cleaning and assembly of stapling units
C. saving time and confusion by knowing the technique of loading the cartridge and anvil before it is needed
D. firing of staple instruments
E. proper placement of safety locks to prevent premature firing of staples

377. Examples of general surgical instruments are
A. Jameson muscle hook
B. Barraguer needle holder
C. Jaeger retractor
D. McPherson speculum
E. none of the above

378. The Cushing elevator is most often used for
A. eye surgery
B. nasal surgery
C. neurosurgery
D. cardiovascular surgery
E. none of the above

379. Nasal instruments include
A. the Aufricht retractor
B. Hartmann dressing forceps
C. Joseph "button knife"
D. Grieshaber trephine
E. all of the above

380. Instrumentation for knee surgery would include
A. Stille-Luer rongeur
B. Bennett retractors
C. osteotomes
D. short curettes
E. Loman bone clamp

381. Patients themselves are a source of contamination to their open wound. Contamination can occur from
A. circulating blood
B. respiratory tract
C. GI tract
D. skin
E. all of the above

382. Members of the scrub team are a potent source of contamination to the surgical wound. Efforts to minimize this source include

A. proper ventilation within the OR

• B. scrubbing, gowning, and gloving

• C. covering all exposed hair

D. use of antiseptic on the patient's skin

• E. not touching the patient's skin with the sterile gloved hand

383. Guidelines for prevention of direct contamination and cross-contamination published in <u>Standards of Practice</u>, published by the Association of Operating Room Nurses, recommend which of the following?

A. Only items that have come in contact with the patient are considered contaminated

• B. Wet vacuum method of OR floor cleaning should be used

• C. Use gloves or instrument when collecting and counting sponges

D. Cleaning OR between cases is considered terminal cleaning

• E. All surgical procedures are treated as contaminated

V

SURGERY

13. SURGICAL PROCEDURES

DIRECTIONS: Each of the questions or incomplete statements below is followed by five suggested answers or completions. Select the most appropriate answer(s).

---

384. The incision used for upper, middle, or lower abdominal procedures can be either on the right or left and is called the
   A. longitudinal midline
   B. hypochondrial
   • C. paramedian rectus
   D. epigastric
   E. midabdominal transverse

385. The vertical midline incision is used for
   • A. gastric cases
   B. all colon cases
   C. gall bladder surgery
   • D. some gynecological cases
   E. all of the above

386. A Pfannenstiel incision will most probably be used for which of the following procedures?
   A. Splenectomy
   B. Gastrectomy
   • C. Hysterectomy
   D. Cholecystectomy
   E. Whipple procedure

387. The McBurney incision is known as the
   A. inverted U incision
   • B. muscle-splitting incision
   • C. lower oblique incision
   • D. appendix incision
   E. none of the above

388. What type of surgery can be performed when the surgeon makes a subcostal incision?
   A. Common bile duct exploration
   B. Cholecystectomy
   C. Splenectomy
   D. A and B
 • E. All of the above

389. The thoracoabdominal incision is used for gastrectomy, splenectomy, and surgery of the lower end of the esophagus. It is made in which of the following areas?
   A. From the side of the umbilicus laterally to the lumbar region at an angle to the crest of the ilium
   B. From a point just below the costal area on one side in the axillary line to the same point on the opposite side
 • C. From a point midway between the xiphoid process and umbilicus, extends over the costal margin to the mid-scapular region
   D. From a point between the xiphoid and umbilicus, extends laterally to a point in the axillary line just below the costal margin
   E. None of the above

390. A well-planned incision would consider the following characteristics
   A. minimum exposure
 • B. ease and speed of closure
 • C. minimum postoperative discomfort
   D. healing by granulation
   E. not easily extended

391. The right upper paramedian incision could be used for
   A. repair of hiatus hernia
   B. sigmoid colon
   C. gastrectomy
   D. appendectomy
 • E. biliary tract surgery

392. Which of the following are true of the lower abdominal midline incision?
 • A. It provides excellent exposure of the pelvic organs
   B. It is stronger than the paramedian incision
   C. It is not easily extended
 • D. It may be used for suprapubic prostatectomy
 • E. It is begun opposite the umbilicus

393. Closure of abdominal wounds includes
- • A. continuous chromic peritoneal stitches
- • B. muscle and fascia closure with interrupted sutures or staples
- C. heavy, continuous, subcutaneous stitches
- D. cutting-edge needles for peritoneum
- • E. silk, nylon, or staples for skin closure

14. GENERAL SURGERY

DIRECTIONS: Each of the questions or incomplete statements below is followed by five suggested answers or completions. Select the most appropriate answer(s).

---

394. A laparotomy is an incision made through the abdominal wall and into the peritoneal cavity. To accomplish this, it is necessary to have
   - • A. suction and counted sponges
   - • B. Richardson and Kelly retractors
   - C. Finochette retractor
   - D. Blake forceps
   - • E. knife handles, 3, 4 and 7

395. Which of the following statements concerning hernias are true?
   - • A. A protrusion of any viscus or tissue through a congenital or acquired opening in the wall of its natural cavity
   - • B. Classified anatomically
   - C. Always have a sac present
   - D. Usually considered a minor problem easily repaired
   - E. Never found in patients under thirty

396. A hernia which cannot be reduced is the
   - • A. Incarcerated hernia
   - B. Diaphragmatic hernia
   - C. Direct inguinal hernia
   - D. Indirect inguinal hernia
   - E. Femoral hernia

397. The most common type of hernias are
- A. femoral
- B. inguinal
- C. umbilical
- D. hiatus
- E. ventral

398. An incarcerated hernia
- A. may or may not cause intestinal obstruction
- B. results in pain in the regional hernia swelling
- C. does not require immediate treatment
- D. is the same as a ventral hernia
- E. all of the above

399. Removal of the entire involved breast without lymph node dissection describes
- A. radical mastectomy
- B. modified radical mastectomy
- C. simple or total mastectomy
- D. partial mastectomy (lumpectomy)
- E. subcutaneous mastectomy

400. Excising a portion of a breast mass for pathological examination describes
- A. excisional biopsy
- B. needle biopsy
- C. incisional biopsy
- D. incision and drainage
- E. none of the above

401. Diagnostic techniques for detection of early breast disease include
- A. mammography
- B. thermography
- C. ultrasound
- D. physical exams
- E. all of the above

402. Operative procedure following incisional breast biopsy with immediate diagnosis indicating further surgery may require
   - A. closure of the biopsy incision with continuous locking sutures
   - B. removal of the biopsy instruments
   - C. change of gown and gloves
   - D. reprepping and redraping of the operative site
   - •E. all of the above

403. If varicose veins are clinically diagnosed and surgery indicated
   - •A. insufficiency of deep femoral veins should be ruled out
   - •B. OR preparation will extend from lower abdomen to ankles
   - •C. skin incisions are made in the groin and ankle
   - D. minor dressings are applied on all incisions
   - E. only the saphenous vein is involved

404. Rectal surgery
   - A. is usually performed in the lithotomy position
   - B. is always performed under general anesthesia
   - •C. may require use of dye or probes and grooved director
   - •D. may use electrocautery or cryosurgery
   - E. all of the above

405. A direct inguinal hernia
   - A. protrudes into the inguinal canal through the internal ring
   - B. protrudes between the internal and external oblique muscles
   - •C. protrudes directly through the transversalis fascia below the deep epigastric vessels
   - •D. emerges at the external inguinal ring
   - E. none of the above

406. The veins most commonly involved in varicosities are
   - A. posterior tibial
   - B. femoral
   - •C. saphenous
   - D. anterior tibial
   - E. basilic

407. Varicosities can be repaired by
- • A. a simple spot removal, by ligation above the distention, and excision
- • B. a procedure where an external stripper is slipped over the cut end of the vein and removes all branches and surrounding tissues and an internal stripper is inserted into the lumen of the vessel and pushed down until obstruction is reached and removed
- C. excision of all anterior veins in leg
- D. excision of all posterior veins in leg
- E. none of the above

408. A hemorrhoidectomy
- • A. is a ligation and excision of a dilated vein
- B. is an incision and draining procedure
- • C. usually requires a transfixion suture placed in the mucosa
- • D. can be an excision and evacuation of external thrombosed area
- E. none of the above

15. GENERAL ABDOMINAL SURGERY

DIRECTIONS: Each of the questions or incomplete statements below is followed by five suggested answers or completions. Select the most appropriate answer(s).

409. Which of the following statements are valid concerning an appendectomy?
   A. If extensive pathology is not suspected, a McBurney incision is made
   B. The appendix is attached to the ileum and, therefore, additional bowel instruments should be available in case an ileostomy needs to be done
   C. When the appendix has ruptured, the peritoneal cavity is usually drained
   D. A purse string suture is always used
   E. A sponge count is not required

410. A cholecystectomy
   A. can be performed through a right subcostal incision or right paramedian incision
   B. can be performed through a left subcostal or paramedian incision
   C. requires that the cystic duct and artery be divided, ligated, and transfixed with suture
   D. requires that the common bile duct be identified and not injured
   E. requires that the common bile duct be divided and ligated

411. An obstruction in the biliary system may be caused by tumor, stricture, or inflammatory lesions. The surgical procedure to relieve this problem could be
   A. cholecystojejunostomy
   B. choledochojejunostomy
   C. cholecystoduodenostomy
   D. choledochoduodenostomy
   • E. any of the above

412. What suture might the surgeon choose to sew the gall bladder bed?
   A. 0 chromic—large taper needle
   B. 3-0 plain—large taper needle
   C. 4-0 silk—straight cutting needle
   • D. 3-0 chromic—small taper needle
   E. 1 chromic—small taper needle

413. Cholecystectomy with cholangiogram is scheduled. What supplies are necessary?
   A. Observe that circulating nurse has OR table with x-ray cassette
   B. Radiopaque dye (hypaque), cholangiogram catheters, syringes
   C. Bakes dilators, probes, scoops
   D. Assorted sizes of T tubes
   • E. All of the above

414. Strictures of the common and hepatic ducts may be repaired by
   • A. resection of stricture with end-to-end anastomosis over a T tube
   B. aspiration of the duct
   • C. anastomosis between the duct or ducts and the intestines
   D. grafting of the duct
   E. all of the above

415. A Whipple procedure is
   A. considered a radical procedure
   B. usually done because of cancer of the head of the pancreas
   C. removal of the head of the pancreas, the entire duodenum, a portion of the jejunum, the distal third of the stomach, the lower half of the common bile duct, and a portion of the pancreatic duct
   D. also known as pancreaticoduodenectomy
   • E. all of the above

416. When a hepatic resection is scheduled, a biopsy could be taken, a tumor removed, or a lobectomy performed. To meet all possibilities, what should the ORT (operating room technologist) have available?
   A. Manometer to check pressure
   B. Special suture
   C. Chest instruments if surgeon decides to use throaco-abdominal approach
   D. Electrocautery
   E. All of the above

417. Anastomosis in the area of the GI tract
   A. requires no special equipment or technique
   B. requires use of bowel technique
   C. always requires changing of gloves and drapes after resection and anastomosis
   D. none of the above
   E. all of the above

418. Which of the following conditions might cause an esophageal obstruction?
   A. Infection
   B. Swallowing a caustic substance, such as lye
   C. Foreign body
   D. Tumor
   E. All of the above

419. The procedure to reconstruct the area between the stomach and the duodenum is called
   A. gastrotomy
   B. pylorotomy
   C. pyloroplasty
   D. pyloromyotomy
   E. none of the above

420. Implantable devices such as the Hickman catheter or infusaid pump may be necessary for the following
   A. chemotherapy
   B. pain relief
   C. nutritional support
   D. infection control
   E. all of the above

421. Which of the following instruments and supplies would NOT be necessary for the appendectomy procedure?
   A. Straight hemostats and Babcocks
   B. Chromic 2-0 suture on a GI needle
   C. Richardson and Parker retractors
   D. Single-tooth tenaculum
   E. Heaney forceps

422. When the common duct is opened in biliary surgery
   A. the Ochsner trocar may be used
   B. care must be exercised to isolate instruments used
   C. drains are usually not necessary
   D. aspiratory needle and syringe may assist in identification of the duct
   E. x-rays are not required

423. Which is NOT true of choledochoscopy?
   A. It may be used instead of operative cholangiogram
   B. It requires the use of the choledochoscope and accessories
   C. It is indirect visualization of the bile ducts
   D. It does not require abdominal opening
   E. It requires copious amounts of irrigating saline

424. Causes for splenectomy include
   A. hypersplenism
   B. traumatic rupture
   C. accessory spleen
   D. tumors
   E. all of the above

425. Which is NOT true of splenectomy?
   A. A thoracoabdominal incision may be used
   B. The abdomen is often filled with blood
   C. Right angle, vascular, and pedicle clamps may be used
   D. Mayo and Allen clamps are used
   E. Heavy silk is used to tie and ligate vessels

426. Parietal cell vagotomy is often the preferred treatment for
   A. carcinoma of the pancreas
   B. morbid obesity
   C. chronic duodenal ulcer
   D. Crohn's disease
   E. esophageal varices

427. Partial gastrectomy with gastroduodenostomy performed for chronic gastric ulcer, perforating ulcer, or tumor would require
- A. Allis or Babcock clamps
- B. Kocher and Allen clamps
- C. silk sutures or stapling instruments
- D. colostomy rod
- E. ligature carriers

428. The gastric bypass, gastroplasty, or gastric partioning procedures are performed for
- A. Crohn's disease
- B. pancreatitis
- C. morbid obesity
- D. gastric ulcer
- E. none of the above

429. The Koch pouch ileostomy procedure
- A. is a surgically constructed intestinal reservoir
- B. follows a proctocolectomy in a one-stage operation
- C. creates a stoma site usually in the right lower quadrant
- D. is obsolete
- E. none of the above

430. An ileostomy is done
- A. for intestinal obstruction
- B. for strangulated intestines
- C. when a total colectomy is contemplated
- D. when the appendix ruptures
- E. none of the above

431. Regarding a colostomy, an opening made into the transverse or descending colon
- A. it is always permanent
- B. it can be done to give rest to the colon
- C. it is impossible to close again
- D. all of the above
- E. none of the above

432. An abdominoperineal resection is done because of
- A. cancer of the cecum
- B. cancer of the hepatic flexure of the colon
- C. ulcerative colitis
- D. Meckel's diverticulum
- E. malignant lesions of the lower sigmoid colon, rectum, and anus

16. EAR, NOSE, MOUTH, AND THROAT SURGERY

DIRECTIONS: Each of the questions or incomplete statements below is followed by five suggested answers or completions. Select the most appropriate answer(s).

---

433. A submucous resection is
   - A. performed strictly for cosmetic purposes
   - B. the removal of portions of the septum
   - C. done to relieve nasal polyps
   - D. performed when an injury, deformity, or fracture of the septum interferes with normal respiratory function
   - E. all of the above

434. What instruments would you pick for a submucous resection?
   - A. Cartilage knife, bayonet forceps
   - B. Freer elevator, Frazier suction tip
   - C. Small osteotomes, mallet
   - D. Nasal saws, double-action nasal rongeur
   - E. All of the above

435. Procedures done on the sinuses are
   - A. intra-nasal antrostomy
   - B. removal of nasal polyps
   - C. Caldwell-Luc (radial antrostomy)
   - D. ethmoidectomy
   - E. all of the above

436. What instruments are necessary in order to perform a tonsillectomy and adenoidectomy?
   - A. Jennings or McIvor mouth gag
   - B. Adenoid curettes
   - C. Schnitz or tonsil hemostat
   - D. Yankauer suction
   - E. All of the above

437. Procedures on the thyroid gland require a basic dissecting set of instruments plus
    A. Lahey forceps vulsellum
    B. Green retractors, Farr or spring retractors
    C. self-retaining thyroid retractor
    D. straight and curved fine hemostats
    E. all of the above

438. During a thyroidectomy, what structures does the surgeon always identify?
    A. Larynx
    B. Parathyroid glands
    C. Recurrent laryngeal nerve
    D. Jugular vein
    E. Hypoglossal duct

439. Parotidectomy is done for removal of benign and malignant tumors, for inflammatory lesions, and for vascular anomalies. During this procedure the surgeon needs to preserve certain tissues, so he must
    A. identify the auricular nerve
    B. identify the superficial temporal artery and vein
    C. identify the external jugular vein
    D. identify the temporal, zygomatic, mandibular, and cervical branches of the facial nerve
    E. all of the above

440. What instruments and supplies would be necessary for laryngectomy and radical neck dissection?
    A. Bone-cutting forceps, rongeur, Gigli saws, possibly a Stryker saw
    B. Osteotomes, periosteal elevators, mallet
    C. Bovie suction, Frazier suction
    D. Laryngectomy tubes, multiple mosquito clamps
    E. All of the above

441. Equipment and instruments needed for mastoidectomy would include
    A. rongeur, Proud fascia crusher, House endaural retractor
    B. endaural curettes
    C. Jordan Day drill, Wullstein drill with burrs
    D. Bishop-Harmon forceps, VonGriffe fixation forceps, Castroviejo forceps
    E. none of the above

442. Simple mastoidectomy is the
   A. removal of the bony osseous wall dividing the meatus from the antrum and attic
   B. destruction of the middle ear
   C. removal of the air cells of the mastoid process without disturbing the contents of the middle ear
   D. most common treatment of otitis media
   E. none of the above

443. Septorhinoplasty
   A. involves a skin graft
   B. is performance of a septoplasty and rhinoplasty together
   C. restores both cosmetic appearance and function
   D. requires packing of the sinuses
   E. may extract a mucocele

444. The terms septoplasty, septal reconstruction, and submucous resection
   A. are used interchangeably
   B. all refer to correction of a deviated septum
   C. describe the creation of a patent airway and straight septal line
   D. describe the creation of a nasoantral window
   E. include the removal of the inferior turbinates

445. Regarding tracheotomy tubes
   A. most are disposable and come in a variety of styles and sizes
   B. they must be available in the set-up before the trachea is incised
   C. they have an attached cuff that must be tested for leakage
   D. they can become dislodged from the trachea if not airtight
   E. all of the above

446. Which of the following would NOT be included on the tracheotomy set-up?
   A. Biopsy forcep
   B. Trousseau dilator
   C. Tracheal hook
   D. Tracheotomy tape
   E. Pole retractors

447. Treatment for hyperparathyroidism, parathyroidectomy, or removal of parathyroid adenoma involves
   - A. identification and isolation of recurrent laryngeal nerve
   - B. incision of deep cervical fascia
   - C. rapid dissection
   - D. heavy catgut suture
   - E. removal of one gland

448. The use of lasers, first applied in otalaryngology, is advantageous
   - A. for excision of polyps on the larynx
   - B. because it provides hemostasis and simultaneous cauterization
   - C. because all laser equipment is the same
   - D. because this equipment is inexpensive
   - E. because it does not require any special safety precautions

449. Precautions when using the laser include
   - A. wrapping the endotracheal tube
   - B. wearing of glasses by all OR personnel
   - C. moist gauze to protect the patient's eyes
   - D. moist neurosurgical patties through the laryngoscope
   - E. all of the above

450. Which of the following is NOT a type of implantable ear prosthetic?
   - A. Hall micro-ototome
   - B. Vein (polyethylene) strut
   - C. Disposable myringotomy tubes
   - D. Teflon wire
   - E. Stainless steel piston

451. Tympanoplasty
   - A. restores or improves hearing of patients with middle ear hearing loss
   - B. is the reconstruction of the tympanic membranes often accomplished by means of a vein graft
   - C. requires microscope, drill, burrs, dissectors, suction, and bovie
   - D. is usually performed under local anesthesia
   - E. A and C

452. Regarding myringotomy
   A. it is the cutting of the tympanic membrane visualized by the microscope
   B. it is a treatment for acute otitis media
   C. instrument set-up needed includes myringotomy knife, Noyes needle, ear speculum, suction tips, forceps, eustachian tube prosthesis
   D. culture may be taken to determine causative organisms of infection
   • E. all of the above

453. Regarding stapedectomy
   • A. it is the removal of stapes and reestablishment of linkage between the incus and oval window
   • B. it restores hearing in patients with conductive deafness
   C. it is considered minor surgery
   • D. it usually requires a vein graft, polyethylene tube, or other prosthetic material
   E. it does not require the use of the microscope

17. OPHTHALMIC SURGERY

DIRECTIONS: Each of the questions or incomplete statements below is followed by five suggested answers or completions. Select the most appropriate answer(s).

---

454. Examples of intraocular procedures are
   - A. cataract extraction
   - B. removal of pterygium
   - C. scleral buckling of retinal detachment
   - D. ptosis repair
   - E. entropian repair

455. Corneal transplant (penetrating keratoplasty) requires
   - A. enucleation of the recipient
   - B. trephination of the donor and recipient corneas
   - C. anastomosis of the recti and inferior oblique muscles
   - D. use of a cryoextractor
   - E. protection of the eye with a Fox shield

456. Which would be important for the ORT to consider in preparing for the scleral buckling procedure?
   - A. Surgical preparation of the eye is not necessary
   - B. Implants should be rinsed in saline
   - C. Four rectus muscles of the eye will be isolated and tagged with suture
   - D. Diathermy and transilluminator will be used
   - E. None of the above

457. To obtain appropriate specimens for the eye bank
   - A. eyes are removed immediately after death
   - B. special consent forms are required
   - C. aseptic conditions are not required
   - D. eyes are placed in specimen bottles with the cornea down
   - E. all of the above

458. Regarding the phacoemulsification or phacofragmentation method of cataract extraction
   A. it requires extensive suturing
   B. it requires a long convalescence
   C. an activated needle breaks up the lens with ultrasonic vibration
   D. it is an intracapsular extraction
   E. irrigation-aspiration flow removes fragments

459. Vitrectomy is performed for
   A. vitreal opacities
   B. vitreal hemorrhage
   C. prolapse of the iris
   D. conjunctival laceration
   E. certain types of retinal detachment

460. Photocoagulation
   A. is used to treat a retinal tear or hole not surrounded by detachment
   B. utilizes an intense source of multiwavelength light (xenon tube)
   C. is the same as laser treatment
   D. is delivered by the direct ophthalmoscope
   E. requires the use of special glasses

461. The intraocular lens (IOL)
   A. allows the patient almost immediate postoperative vision
   B. is manufactured in many forms
   C. is inserted following cataract extraction
   D. requires preparation with neutralizing solution at the time of implant
   E. all of the above

462. Instruments and supplies needed for the filtering procedure for glaucoma include
   A. cryoextractor
   B. Bishop-Harmon forceps and tenotomy scissors
   C. 6-0 to 9-0 silk or nylon
   D. Burch pick
   E. all of the above

463. Surgery for strabismus is known as
- A. resection and recession procedure
- B. scleral buckling
- C. phacoemulsification
- D. enucleation
- E. evisceration of the eye

464. Instruments needed on an eye muscle procedure are
- A. lid speculum, muscle hooks
- B. caliper
- C. Steven scissors, Castroviejo forceps and needle holder
- D. DeBakey forceps
- E. Glassman clamps

465. Which of the following statements are NOT true concerning cataract extraction?
- A. Two methods are used—intracapsular or extra-capsular
- B. Transfixation suture is usually used; 4-0 silk may be the choice
- C. Cautery is not routinely included on set-up, as the eye is avascular
- D. Iridectomy is performed; the lens is grasped and removed with a cryoextractor
- E. Lens may be grasped and removed with a cryo-extractor

466. Iridectomy is the removal of iris tissue. This is usually done for
- A. cataracts
- B. treatment of some cases of acute glaucoma
- C. reestablishment of communication between posterior and anterior chambers in order to establish a flow of aqueous fluid
- D. the establishing of drainage paths to lacrimal ducts
- E. none of the above

467. Surgery to treat retinal separation (detachment) could be
- A. diathermy
- B. iridectomy
- C. cryosurgery
- D. scleral buckling
- E. iridencleisis

18. PLASTIC AND RECONSTRUCTIVE SURGERY

DIRECTIONS: Each of the questions or incomplete statements below is followed by five suggested answers or completions. Select the most appropriate answer(s).

---

468. Skin grafts are classified
    A. composite
    B. split thickness
    C. flaps
    D. full thickness
    • E. all of the above

469. When a pedicle flap graft is created, it consists of skin and subcutaneous tissue of the donor site and
    A. is left attached to the donor site
    B. is sutured directly to the recipient site
    C. supplies blood to areas to be grafted
    D. may be immobilized during healing
    • E. all of the above

470. Most esthetic surgery is classified as plastic/ reconstructive surgery. Some examples would be
    • A. dermabrasion
    B. electrolysis
    • C. rhinoplasty
    • D. blepharoplasty
    E. all of the above

471. Regarding cleft lip, a condition where the lip does not fuse as the embryo matures
    A. it can be corrected by different methods of suturing
    • B. its cause is unknown
    • C. it usually occurs in 1 out of 750 births
    • D. it is usually corrected at age 3 or 4 months
    E. it is usually corrected after the age of 7 years

472. Cleft palate
    A. is usually corrected 6 weeks after birth
    B. allows food and liquid to escape into the nasal cavity
    C. is usually repaired at 18-24 months of age
    D. will require the use of orthodontics following repair
    E. does not affect speech

473. Rhytidectomy is
    A. plastic repair of the nose
    B. excision of excessively wrinkled skin of the face and chin
    C. accomplished through incision and undermining of the skin
    D. performed under general as well as local anesthesia
    E. all of the above

474. Plastic and reconstructive surgery often requires the use of skin graft or skin flaps. To determine which type of cover would be used depends on
    A. size of defect
    B. blood supply
    C. quality of the skin surrounding the defect
    D. location of defect
    E. all of the above

475. What might be substituted for sterile marking pens?
    A. Regular ball point pen
    B. Needle
    C. Electrocautery
    D. Wooden applicator and dye
    E. Skin hook

476. Dermabrasion may be employed to
    A. remove scars of trauma or acne
    B. remove tattoos
    C. treat microtia
    D. remove excess skin around the eyes
    E. control hemorrhage

477. Erich or Jelenko splint refers to
    A. an operation for reshaping the nose
    B. lip reconstruction
    C. reshaping of the chin
    D. method of fixation in fractures of the mandible and maxilla
    E. transfacial nerve grafting

478. Which of the following is NOT true of the Brown or Hall dermatomes?
   A. Have adjustable depth gauges
   B. Do not limit the length of the graft
   C. Consist of one-half of a metal drum
   D. Utilize a dermatome tape
   E. May be electrical or air powered

479. Methods of stent fixation to obtain pressure are
   A. long suture ends tied crisscross over a dressing
   B. used when an area cannot be bandaged snugly
   C. prosthetic implants
   D. fine mesh gauze
   E. taping a form-fitting mold over the nose

480. Breast reconstruction after mastectomy
   A. is not delayed by chemotherapy and/or radiation therapy
   B. does not include the nipple-areola area
   C. may be a latissimus dorsi myocutaneous island flap
   D. many include a silastic implant
   E. interferes with detecting recurrences of disease

481. Reduction mammoplasty
   A. is the same as augmentation mammoplasty
   B. may be indicated for ptosis
   C. may be indicated if back pain and poor posture result from large breasts
   D. utilizes silicone implants
   E. is a procedure for gynecomastia

19. GYNECOLOGY

DIRECTIONS: Each of the questions or incomplete statements below is followed by five suggested answers or completions. Select the most appropriate answer(s).

---

482. A radical vulvectomy and groin lymphadenectomy is
    A. the removal of the labia majora and minora
    B. done to treat intractable pruritis
    C. the dissection of skin of the abdomen and groin, labia majora and minora, clitoris, mons pubis and portions of urethra, and vagina plus superficial and deep inguinal nodes
    D. a procedure which can have a psychological effect on the patient
    E. all of the above

483. A vaginal plastic or anterior/posterior repair operation is done
    A. to relieve stress incontinence
    B. to repair a cystocele
    C. to repair a rectocele
    D. to repair an enterocele
    E. all of the above

484. Myomectomy is
    A. done for malignancy
    B. done on women of child-bearing age
    C. the removal of benign growth from muscle wall of uterus
    D. performed routinely by a vaginal approach
    E. none of the above

485. A pelvic exenteration is
   A. a radical procedure
   B. the removal of all pelvic organs
   C. the excision of lymph nodes and chains
   D. usually an abdominoperineal procedure
   E. all of the above

486. If a patient has experienced a ruptured tubal pregnancy, which of the following procedures may be performed?
   A. Salpingectomy
   B. Oophorectomy
   C. Trying to save the ovary, a wedge resection may be done
   D. A panhysterectomy
   E. None of the above

487. A Marshall-Marchetti operation is
   A. performed to treat urinary incontinence and uterine prolapse
   B. performed to repair muscle tears of the pelvic floor
   C. performed to repair a protrusion of the cul-de-sac of Douglas
   D. another name for an anterior, posterior repair
   E. a simple vulvectomy

488. Laparoscopy is endoscopic visualization of the peritoneal cavity through the anterior abdominal wall. Laparoscopy
   A. provides the gynecologist the same anatomical view of the pelvic organs as seen at the diagnostic laparotomy
   B. enables procedures such as aspiration of cysts, lysis of adhesions, tissue biopsies, and sterilization to be performed
   C. may enable the surgeon to avoid unnecessary pelvic surgery
   D. can only be performed after establishment of a pneumoperitoneum
   E. all of the above

489. When a laparoscopy is performed, what gas is instilled into the abdominal cavity via the Verres needle?
   A. Carbon dioxide
   B. Carbon monoxide
   C. Nitrous oxide
   D. Nitrogen
   E. Oxygen

490. Cesarean section is delivery of an infant through abdominal incision. Abdominal instruments are needed, plus
   . A. bandage scissors, bulb syringe
   . B. Pennington clamps or small ring forceps, Pitocin, suction, bovie
   C. Heaney clamps, uterine sound, and single and double-toothed tenaculum
   .D. delivery forceps should be available
   E. Somer clamp

491. Besides the routine two sponge counts which occur in a laparotomy, when is the additional sponge count taken during a cesarean section?
   A. There is no additional sponge count taken
   B. There are usually two more counts taken, immediately after the baby and placenta have been delivered
   . C. As the uterus is being closed
   D. At the time of peritonealization
   E. As fascia is being closed

492. Suction curettage
   A. is performed for cervical biopsy
   B. requires extensive dilatation of the cervix
   . C. is performed for early termination of pregnancy
   . D. provides less chance for uterine perforation
   E. all of the above

493. Which of the following would NOT be used for uterine dilatation?
   A. Hegar dilators
   . B. Jackson retractor
   . C. Gaylor forceps
   D. Goodell dilator
   E. Hank dilators

494. Which of the following are NOT methods of biopsy and conization of the cervix?
   . A. Cesium insertion
   B. Scalpel and suturing
   C. Use of the laser
   . D. Shirodkar operation
   E. Application of electrocautery

495. Causes for uterine suspension include
   A. pelvic inflammatory disease or endometriosis
   B. tuboplasty
   C. treatment of symptoms of uterine retroversion
   D. malignant tumor
   E. none of the above

496. Success of tubal ligation reversal may depend on extent of tubal destruction. Methods of tubal ligation include
   A. laparoscopy
   B. Falope ring
   C. cauterization
   D. Pomeroy technique
   E. microsurgery

497. Surgical hazards of the hysterectomy procedure include
   A. injury to the ureters
   B. injury to the bladder
   C. injury to the bowel
   D. hemorrhage
   E. all of the above

498. In the cesarean section procedure, suction is imperative
   A. when opening the peritoneum
   B. once the membranes are excised
   C. to develop the bladder flap
   D. when the abdominal incision is made
   E. when the cord is clamped

20. GENITOURINARY SURGERY

DIRECTIONS: Each of the questions or incomplete statements below is followed by five suggested answers or completions. Select the most appropriate answer(s).

---

499. A cystoscope is required for visual inspection of the bladder and adjacent structures. The necessary and accessory parts of a cystoscope which allow the best possible vision are
    - A. the operating telescope
    - B. single and double catheterizing telescopes
    - C. concave and convex sheaths
    - D. obturator, electrode post, cord, and power source
    - · E. all of the above

500. Whenever there is an interruption into the urinary tract, there is a danger of leakage of urine. Special draining tubes would include
    - · A. Foley catheter
    - B. Pilcher bag
    - · C. Malecot or Pezzer catheter
    - · D. Robinson catheter
    - E. all of the above

501. Nephrectomy is removal of a kidney. The routine set-up for this procedure would include
    - A. gastrointestinal instruments
    - · B. rib shears, elevators, and strippers
    - · C. Mixter clamps
    - D. Demartel clamp
    - · E. Young pedicle clamp

502. A cystometer is used to
   A. measure the depth of the bladder
   B. give the level of elasticity of the urethra
   C. assess the pressure response of the bladder to distention
   D. note bladder capacity
   E. evaluate neurogenic dysfunction

503. A pyeloureteroplasty would need the instrument set-up for nephrectomy, plus
   A. small Schnidt gall duct forceps
   B. Iris scissors
   C. small Metzenbaum scissors
   D. mosquito clamps
   E. all of the above

504. A kidney transplant requires routine equipment and instruments for the donor nephrectomy. The special equipment needed on the set-up for the recipient would include
   A. clip applicators
   B. vascular instruments
   C. fine suture material
   D. tubes for a cystotomy drain
   E. all of the above

505. In order for a patient to be dialyzed, there must be an arteriovenous access. This is
   A. called an AV fistula
   B. a Scribner shunt with a visible cannula system
   C. a procedure which can be done under local anesthesia
   D. a procedure always done under general anesthesia
   E. a high-risk procedure

506. An ileal conduit
   A. is usually made with a 15-20 cm-segment of terminal ileum, a few inches from the ileocecal valve
   B. is a procedure where care must be exercised in ligation of mesenteric vessels to preserve the ileocecal artery
   C. is a procedure where only dissection is carried out without anastomosis
   D. creates a stoma
   E. all of the above

507. A cystectomy is
   A. a simple, routine procedure
   B. done only for malignancy or congenital damage causing nonfunction
   C. a procedure that requires ureteral transplant
   D. considered a radical procedure
   E. none of the above

508. Partial or total adrenalectomy is done
   A. routinely if adrenals are damaged during surgery
   B. to control hormone secretions in some conditions of carcinoma
   C. to lower blood pressure
   D. to treat adrenal hyperfunction
   E. to remove tumor

509. For unilateral adrenalectomy, the patient may be put in supine or lateral position. For a bilateral exploration of adrenals, the patient is usually
   A. placed in Sims position
   B. placed in prone position
   C. placed in supine position
   D. placed in lateral position
   E. none of the above

510. A prostatectomy is usually performed because
   A. the prostate is causing urinary obstruction
   B. the patient desires sterilization
   C. of benign hypertrophy
   D. of malignancy
   E. all of the above

511. Special equipment needed in an abdominal prostatectomy procedure includes
   A. vascular instruments
   B. a Lowsley forceps
   C. urethral sounds
   D. Iris scissors
   E. a Lowsley tractor

512. A prostatectomy can be performed by different methods, such as
   A. suprapubic
   B. perineal
   C. retropubic
   D. transurethral
   E. all of the above

513. Reconstruction of the vas
    A. is impossible
    B. is never attempted
    C. is done by microsurgical repair
    D. requires excision of scar tissue to open the lumen of the vas
    E. all of the above

514. Orchiectomy (removal of testes)
    A. controls hormone secretion in malignancy
    B. relieves obstruction
    C. removes damaged organs from trauma or atrophy
    D. may be indicated following infection
    E. all of the above

515. Insertion of the penile prosthesis is usually done
    A. as a treatment for impotence
    B. in the supine position
    C. with the rigid, small, carrion-type prosthesis
    D. with the Scott inflatable prosthesis
    E. all of the above

516. Coagulum pyelolithotomy
    A. is used for removal of large renal calculi
    B. usually requires an abdominal incision
    C. is a method to remove multiple calculi from the renal collecting system
    D. necessitates intraoperative pyelogram
    E. utilizes a fibrinogen, thrombin, calcium chloride mixture

517. Common vascular access procedures for hemodialysis may include
    A. venous catheterization
    B. arteriovenous shunts
    C. bovine graft
    D. arteriovenous fistula
    E. all of the above

518. Considerations for hydrocelectomy procedure include
    A. lithotomy position
    B. abdominal incision
    C. moist sponges to prevent painful, postoperative swelling
    D. meticulous hemostasis
    E. application of scrotal support

519. Which of the following, would NOT be a test to evaluate hematuria?
   A. Renal arteriography
   B. Cystoscopy and retrograde pyelography
   C. Computerized axial tomography
   D. Hematological studies
   E. Cystometrogram

520. The donor nephrectomy procedure for kidney transplant requires
   A. a venous catheter
   B. sterile IV tubing
   C. cold saline and electrolyte solution
   D. mosquito clamps
   E. all of the above

521. Which incision is common for the kidney transplant recipient?
   A. Flank
   B. Midline
   C. Curved lower quadrant
   D. Thoracoabdominal
   E. None of the above

522. Considerations for the ileal loop diversion
   A. may be in conjunction with removal of the bladder
   B. selection of a segment of terminal ileum for the ileal conduit
   C. creation of a stoma
   D. none of the above
   E. is the same as vesicostomy

21. THORACIC SURGERY

DIRECTIONS: Each of the questions or incomplete statements below is followed by five suggested answers or completions. Select the most appropriate answer(s).

---

523. Water seal draining is used on cases where the thorax is opened
    A. to provide adequate drainage
    B. to provide draining by suction
    • C. to remove air from the cavity
    • D. to remove serous fluid from the cavity
    E. none of the above

524. Special instruments for surgery on the thoracic cavity would include
    • A. Alexander periosteotome
    B. Hibb's retractors
    • C. Doyen raspatories
    • D. Finochietto retractor
    • E. Bailey contractor

525. Surgical procedures involving removal of lung tissue are
    • A. wedge resection
    B. decortication
    • C. segmental resection
    D. thoracoplasty
    E. thoracentesis

526. Thoracoplasty is the resecting of ribs. This procedure is done
    • A. to produce pulmonary collapse
    • B. to correct a deformed chest
    • C. sometimes in the treatment of tuberculosis
    D. in the treatment of pneumonia
    E. none of the above

527. A pneumonectomy, segmental resection, or lobectomy requires special instruments, such as
   A. Duval forceps
   B. Rummel forceps
   C. Iris scissors
   D. Hudson forceps
   E. Overholt retractor

528. Sternal fractures
   A. cause little disability
   B. can cause problems if ribs are fractured
   C. may have to be pinned or wired
   D. should be repaired, if needed, for thoracic cage stability
   E. all of the above

529. Specimens are obtained through a fiberoptic bronchoscope by
   A. washings
   B. brushings
   C. biopsy forceps
   D. needle biopsy
   E. none of the above

530. Lateral or supine positions may be used for thoracic surgery. Considerations when positioning the patient for thoracic surgery include
   A. avoid abrupt changes to prevent hypotension
   B. provide efficient ventilatory and circulatory functions
   C. median sternotomy gives access to all surfaces of the lung
   D. position does not affect blood return to the heart
   E. all of the above

531. Which procedures would NOT remove a portion of the lung?
   A. Wedge resection
   B. Segmental resection
   C. Pneumonectomy
   D. Lobectomy
   E. Open lung biopsy

532. Which of the following is NOT true of bronchoscopy?
   A. May use a flexible or rigid scope
   B. May be performed to obtain a biopsy
   C. May be used to diagnose esophageal cancer
   D. Allows cultures to be obtained
   E. Requires a light source

533. When collecting bronchoscopy washings
   A. attachment of proper collection bottle to suction is required
   B. specimen container must be held in the upright position
   C. saline may be injected through the scope
   D. an adaptor is required for the endotracheal tube
   E. a flexible brush may be used

534. Mediastinoscopy
   A. allows direct visualization of lymph nodes in the mediastinum
   B. may precede exploratory thoracotomy
   C. does not require incision
   D. is performed under local anesthesia
   E. does not require a light source

535. Reapproximation of the ribs is accomplished with which instrument and heavy catgut suture?
   A. Thoracic stapler
   B. Osteotomes
   C. Alexander
   D. Bailey rib contractor
   E. Bone hook

536. The thoracic stapler may be used
   A. to suture pulmonary vessels
   B. to approximate the ribs
   C. to perform a wedge resection
   D. to suture the bronchus
   E. to stimulate growth of adhesions between the pleurae

537. Groups of lymph nodes of the superior mediastinum that are examined for presence of malignancy via the mediastinoscope include
   A. intrapulmonary
   B. bronchopulmonary
   C. subcarinal or bifurcation nodes
   D. superior tracheobronchial
   E. paratracheal

22. CARDIOVASCULAR SURGERY

DIRECTIONS: Each of the questions or incomplete statements below is followed by five suggested answers or completions. Select the most appropriate answer(s).

---

538. Surgery on the heart requires a variety of special equipment, among which would be
    A. a hypothermia unit
    B. a pump oxygenator
    C. a cardiac monitor and EKG machine
    D. monitoring devices for venous pressure
    E. all of the above

539. Special cardiovascular instruments would include
    A. Satinsky clamps
    B. Harken clamps
    C. Craaford clamps
    D. Potts clamps
    E. all of the above

540. Cardiac catheterization is done
    A. only on the right side
    B. via a cut into a peripheral vein
    C. under sterile procedures
    D. with a radiopaque catheter
    E. all of the above

541. Pericardectomy is usually done through a
    A. left anterior thoracotomy
    B. sternal-splitting incision
    C. left posterior thoracotomy
    D. right thoracotomy
    E. none of the above

542. A sternotomy can be done by
- A. splitting of the bone
- B. use of Lebshe knife
- C. use of an oscillating saw
- D. the Stryker drill
- E. none of the above

543. Poudrage is
- A. application of sterile talcum powder
- B. used to create adhesions
- C. used to treat repeated spontaneous pneumothorax
- D. a palliative measure used for excessive pleural effusion
- E. all of the above

544. Ventricular septal defect
- A. is a rare condition
- B. is found only in males
- C. is a common congenital defect
- D. produces a heart murmur
- E. none of the above

545. Insertion of a cardiac pacemaker may require
- A. an incision through the thorax into the pericardium
- B. an incision into anterolateral prepectoral portion of the chest
- C. a tunnel through subcutaneous tissues
- D. extracorporeal circulation
- E. all of the above

546. Occlusive disease of the major branches of the aorta is most frequently the result of
- A. stenosis
- B. atherosclerosis
- C. ischemia
- D. turbulence
- E. all of the above

547. Arterial injuries are usually managed surgically by
- A. ligation
- B. end-to-end anastomosis
- C. insertion of prosthetic graft
- D. insertion of venous graft
- E. bypass

548. When an endarterectomy is performed, what is removed?
- . A. Atheromatous obstructive plaque
- B. A malignant tumor of the arterial system
- C. A foreign body
- D. A fixed blood clot
- E. An accumulation of air

549. Regarding pulmonary embolism
- A. it can be a complication of surgery
- B. it originates from veins in lower extremities of pelvis
- C. surgery may include vena cava clipping
- D. a filter procedure may be performed on poor-risk patients
- . E. all of the above

550. Aneurysms were once untreatable, but now they can be managed by surgical means. An aneurysm is
- A. narrowing of a blood vessel
- B. vessels blocked with deposits
- ·C. localized dilation of an artery
- D. diffuse dilation of an artery
- E. none of the above

551. Dissecting aneurysms are
- A. the most common acute catastrophe involving the aorta
- B. more common in persons between 45 and 70
- C. more frequently found in persons with some form of congenital heart disease
- D. medial necrosis of the vessel leading to an intimal tear, followed by a dissecting hematoma
- · E. all of the above

552. A common area for aneurysms to develop is in the
- ·A. ascending aorta
- B. radial artery
- ·C. aortic arch
- ·D. descending aorta
- E. none of the above

553. Special equipment needed in the set-up for a portacaval shunt would include
- ·A. spinal manometer
- B. variety of prosthetic grafts
- · C. three-way stopcocks
- D. local anesthetic supplies
- E. all of the above

554. Arteriovenous shunts are performed on patients needing hemodialysis by means of an "artificial kidney." The set-up for this procedure would include
   A. saline and heparin mixture
   B. Teflon-coated vessel appliances
   C. bulldog vascular clamps
   D. vascular sutures
   E. all of the above

555. Ligation of the vena cava usually is done
   A. with a Teflon clip
   B. to prevent pulmonary embolism
   C. to control esophageal bleeding
   D. to slow circulation to the liver
   E. when anticoagulant therapy fails

556. Extraction of arterial emboli may be accomplished by
   A. flushing
   B. irrigation
   C. a balloon catheter
   D. ligation
   E. none of the above

557. Vascular grafts can be
   A. venous autografts
   B. modified bovine grafts
   C. various textiles
   D. various metals
   E. none of the above

558. Coronary artery bypass graft (CABG) requires
   A. sternotomy incision
   B. saphenous vein excision
   C. cardiopulmonary bypass
   D. local or systemic hypothermia
   E. all of the above

559. The pump oxygenator circulates the blood during open heart surgery. What other effects does it have on the blood?
   A. Perfusion
   B. Oxygenation
   C. Cooling
   D. Filtration
   E. All of the above

560. Where are cannulae placed in order for cardiopulmonary bypass to be accomplished?
   A. Carotid artery
   B. Subclavin artery
   C. Vena cava
   D. Ascending aorta
   E. None of the above

561. To increase blood supply to the heart muscle, what procedure may be performed?
   A. Mitral valve replacement
   B. Coronary artery bypass
   C. Permanent pacemaker
   D. Cardiac catheterization
   E. All of the above

562. Kinds of prosthetic heart valves are
   A. biological
   B. anticoagulant
   C. silastic
   D. mechanical
   E. all of the above

563. The first cardiac transplant was performed by Dr. Christian Barnard in 1967. Since that time
   A. heart transplant has steadily increased
   B. distant heart procurement is now possible
   C. immunosuppression is improved with cyclosporin
   D. survival statistics have improved
   E. all of the above

564. Alternatives to mitral valve replacement would include
   A. mitral commissurotomy
   B. angioplasty
   C. mitral annuloplasty
   D. tricuspid valve replacement
   E. all of the above

565. Which would NOT be needed for resection of left ventricular aneurysm?
   A. Cardiopulmonary bypass
   B. Chest tubes
   C. Teflon felt or pledgets
   D. Valve instruments
   E. Prosthetic graft

566. A recent alternative to coronary artery bypass surgery is
   A. permanent pacemaker
   B. coronary angioplasty
   C. aortic balloon
   D. cardiac catheterization
   E. none of the above

567. Placement of transvenous (endocardial) pacing electrodes would require
   A. anterolateral thoracotomy
   B. fluoroscopy
   C. minor instrument set
   D. tunneling instrument
   E. chest tubes

568. Carotid endarterectomy is removal of an atheroma and
   A. may be performed with temporary bypass
   B. may include a patch angioplasty
   C. necessitates clamping of the external, common, and internal carotid arteries
   D. utilizes blunt dissections and Potts Smith angulated scissors
   E. all of the above

23. ORTHOPEDIC SURGERY

DIRECTIONS: Each of the questions or incomplete statements below is followed by five suggested answers or completions. Select the most appropriate answer(s).

---

569. A carposcaphoid fracture is located in the
   A. knee
   B. heel
   . C. wrist
   D. elbow
   E. thumb

570. Colles' fracture is a common type. It involves the
   A. ulna
   . B. radius
   C. femur
   D. tibia
   E. patella

571. Special orthopedic instruments would include
   .A. Bennett retractor
   B. army-navy retractor
   C. Hill retractor
   .D. Lowman holding clamp
   .E. Creggo elevators

572. Arthroplasty of the knee joint usually
   A. requires specially designed instruments for knee operations
   B. is done with the patient's knee flexed
   C. requires use of a tibial plateau prosthesis
   D. is done when the joint appears salvageable
   .E. all of the above

573. If an infection of a bone requires surgery, it involves
   A. introduction of chemicals or drugs
   B. possible decompression of bone and soft tissues
   C. removal of dead bone
   D. debridement of only damaged soft tissue
   E. none of above

574. Exploration or incision into a joint is called
   A. arthrodesis
   B. articulation
   C. arthrotomy
   D. arthroplasty
   E. none of the above

575. The function of the hip may be limited by degenerative lesions such as arthritis. Surgical procedures most commonly used to treat this condition would be
   A. disarticulation
   B. insertion of Moore prosthesis
   C. insertion of metal cup into joint
   D. total hip replacement
   E. none of the above

576. A patellectomy would call for a basic orthopedic set-up plus
   A. Cushing retractors
   B. bone awl
   C. Kocher retractors
   D. fine scissors
   E. all of the above

577. A tibial plateau may be inserted during arthroplasty of the knee joint. Special instruments needed for insertion of the plateau would include
   A. elevators
   B. impactor
   C. strippers
   D. driver
   E. condyle plates

578. Osteogenic sarcoma of a bone when resectable, is usually
   A. a highly malignant tumor
   B. treated by radical amputation
   C. benign
   D. treated by chemotherapy
   E. removed by wide excision

579. Meticulous attention to aseptic technique in orthopedic surgery is critical because
   - • A. infection in bone may cause loss of an extremity
   - • B. operations involve tissues highly susceptible to infection
   - C. operations are performed to correct congenital deformities
   - D. degenerative disease processes are involved
   - E. none of the above

580. Which of the following would be true of orthopedic instrumentation?
   - A. Instruments for hip surgery might be used for hand surgery
   - • B. It may require special care and handling
   - • C. It can be categorized by functional design
   - • D. Cutting instruments require sharpening
   - E. All of the above

581. What can be used for hemostasis in bone?
   - A. Bone cement
   - B. Casts
   - • C. Bone wax
   - D. An allograft
   - E. All of the above

582. What type of suture is usually preferred for periosteum?
   - A. Silk
   - • B. Absorbable
   - C. Nylon
   - D. Wire
   - E. All of the above

583. Nonabsorbable sutures would be used for
   - • A. ligaments
   - • B. muscles
   - C. periosteum
   - • D. tendons
   - E. none of the above

584. A cast should be removed preoperatively to
   - A. allow easier transfer to the OR table
   - B. prevent bone injury
   - C. allow adequate preparation
   - • D. prevent airborne contamination from plaster dust
   - E. facilitate x-ray

585. Which is NOT true of the orthopedic table?
   A. It allows the surgeon to apply traction to a lower extremity while maintaining good alignment and control
   B. It facilitates cast application
   • C. It is the same as the circo-electric bed
   D. It is equipped with various attachments to facilitate x-ray
   • E. It does not require special preparation

586. Why is it recommended that no internal fixation devices be reused?
   A. Galvanic corrosion may occur
   B. Proper identification is not possible
   • C. Scratches, abrasions, and the like affect the strength of an implant
   • D. Imperfections are inevitable with use
   E. Proper cleaning may not be possible

587. Which of the following precautions must be considered when using orthopedic instruments, equipment, and appliances?
   A. Implants must be sterilized according to manufacturer's instructions
   B. Care must be taken to prevent knocking and bumping
   C. Protection can be afforded with special trays and cases
   D. Ultrasonic cleaning should be used if possible
   • E. All of the above

588. Which of the following is NOT true of arthroscopy?
   A. It is a relatively new technique
   • B. Knee flexion is not necessary in the procedure
   C. It allows thorough inspection of every part of the knee through one incision
   D. It provides more variable diagnoses than arthrography
   E. It can employ the use of viewing and recording devices

589. The Bankart procedure involves the
   A. knee
   B. femur
   C. metacarpal joint
   • D. shoulder
   E. radius

24. DIAGNOSTIC PROCEDURES

DIRECTIONS: Each of the questions or incomplete statements below is followed by five suggested answers or completions. Select the most appropriate answer(s).

---

590. Endoscopy refers to the examination of body cavities by means of instruments which permit visual inspection. Usually these procedures are done with topical anesthesia, which would call for use of
   - A. laryngeal mirrors
   - B. endotracheal tube
   - C. spray with straight and curved cannulae
   - D. Jackson forceps
   - E. a syringe with straight and curved cannulae

591. Lymphangiography
   - A. allows visualization of any lymphatic vessel
   - B. requires a fine polyethylene catheter
   - C. is usually done in the OR
   - D. requires general anesthesia
   - E. all of the above

592. Urological fiberoptic instruments differ from other endoscopic fiberoptic equipment in that
   - A. urological instruments are not usually flexible
   - B. the light source is different
   - C. different types of telescopes are used to provide different angle views
   - D. urological instruments are easier to clean
   - E. none of the above

593. Colonoscopy is a common procedure because of increased incidence of colon and rectal cancer. Indications for the procedure include
   A. differential diagnosis of questionable lesions
   B. investigation of lower GI tract bleeding
   C. biopsy of lesions
   D. removal of polypoid lesions
   E. all of the above

594. A procedure to diagnose gastric or duodenal ulcers is
   A. colonoscopy
   B. scleroscopy
   C. esophagoscopy
   D. gastroscopy
   E. none of the above

25. NEUROSURGERY

DIRECTIONS: Each of the questions or incomplete statements below is followed by five suggested answers or completions. Select the most appropriate answer(s).

---

595. Special instruments needed to open the skull would include
   •A. a type of perforator drill
   B. Bethune cutter
   •C. Gigli saws
   •D. self-retaining scalp retractor
   E. Alexander elevator

596. Sponging done during brain surgery must not injure the fragile tissues. The type of sponges usually used are
   A. small gauze compresses
   •B. wet, compressed rayon-cotton pledgets
   C. dry, compressed rayon-cotton pledgets
   D. dry dental rolls
   E. all of the above

597. Exposing instruments for neurosurgical procedures would most frequently include
   A. Weitlaner retractors
   B. vein retractors
   C. dural elevators
   D. mastoid retractors
   •E. all of the above

598. CAT (computerized axial tomography) scanner can be used to
   •A. detect brain tumors
   •B. avoid agonizing diagnostic procedures
   C. register hard data of blood flow
   •D. produce photographs
   E. none of the above

599. Instruments for a craniotomy would include those necessary to open the skull plus a dissecting kit which would contain
   A. bayonet forceps
   B. Oschner clamps (assorted sizes)
   C. spatulas and spoons
   D. small Richardson retractors
   E. assorted aluminum cortex retractors

600. A subdural hematoma may be acute, subacute, or chronic. The acute type requires surgery, usually
   A. within first 2-14 days after injury
   B. within the first 24 hr after injury
   C. evacuation by trephining burr holes
   D. craniotomy
   E. none of the above

601. Percutaneous cordotomy is done on some patients who cannot tolerate open cordotomy for pain relief. This procedure is done
   A. with roentgenographic control
   B. with local anesthesia
   C. with a coagulating needle
   D. as a type of "blind" procedure
   E. all of the above

602. Aneurysms that are intracranial are
   A. outpouchings of the cerebral vessels
   B. usually located deep, at the base of the brain
   C. repaired quickly
   D. thought to be due partly to a congenital defect
   E. none of the above

603. An intracranial aneurysm
   A. is a common abnormality
   B. is found in about 1% of the population
   C. is a "silent" type of lesion
   D. is potentially dangerous, as it can rupture
   E. may impinge on the third nerve or optic chiasm

604. Trigeminal neuralgia (tic douloureux) is a disturbance of the fifth cranial nerve and is characterized by excruciating pain in the face. If it is treated surgically, it is usually by which of the following methods?
   A. Retrogasserian rhizotomy or neurectomy
   B. Lobotomy
   C. Extradural section of the nerve
   D. Electrocoagulation
   E. None of the above

605. Instruments used on surgical procedures of the vertebrae would include
   A. rongeurs, single and double action
   B. Gigli saws
   C. Beckman-Adson retractors
   D. Kerrison rongeurs
   E. Poole suction tip

606. A laminectomy is done for
   A. intractable pain
   B. herniated intervertebral disc
   C. cord tumors
   D. hunchback
   E. compression fracture

607. Hazards of surgery on the vertebrae or spinal cord are
   A. excessive bleeding
   B. sensory nerve damage in lower extremities
   C. complete paraplegia in lower half of body
   D. injury to motor roots resulting in paralysis
   E. none of the above

608. Sympathectomy
   A. commonly is performed to relieve arterial spasm
   B. is done in one specific area of the spinal column
   C. may be performed to increase vascular circulation
   D. always is performed through a flank incision
   E. all of the above

609. Median nerve compression causes nerve palsy in the hand and in some cases is treated surgically by
   A. excision of a portion of the nerve
   B. evulsion at the root
   C. reconstruction of the carpal tunnel
   D. division of the ligament over the course of the nerve
   E. none of the above

610. A frequently performed neurosurgical procedure is laminectomy. Necessary instruments and considerations for this procedure include
   A. basic neurosurgical instrument set
   B. regular cautery and bipolar coagulation units
   C. patient always placed in the prone position
   D. headrest
   E. curettes, rongeurs, periosteal elevators, nerve root retractors

611. Extra concern for control of hemorrhage is important in neurosurgery. Regular and bipolar cautery may be used. The bipolar cautery
   A. has a forcep tip
   B. isolates current output between forcep tips
   C. has a needle tip
   D. requires a grounding pad
   E. none of the above

612. Pituitary rongeurs
   A. facilitate removal of lamina bone
   B. gently move nerves
   C. remove herniated disc material
   D. are all the same size
   E. biopsy brain or tumor tissue

613. Cerebral aneurysm treatment may include
   A. frontotemporal craniotomy
   B. placement of a clip across the base of the lesion
   C. coating with plastic
   D. operating microscope
   E. all of the above

614. For the posterior fossa craniotomy
   A. head shave is not required
   B. prevention of potential air embolism must be considered
   C. sitting position of the patient is usually preferred
   D. a headrest must be used
   E. a single Mayo stand is usually sufficient

615. It is important for the OR technologist to recognize the importance of measures to enhance visibility in neurosurgery. Which of the following are NOT important adjuncts to visibility?
   A. Compressed absorbant patties
   B. Suction
   C. Irrigation
   D. Dura guard attachment
   E. Electrocautery

616. Continuous or intermittent intercranial monitoring may be accomplished by
   A. silicone rubber suction drain
   B. subarachnoid screw
   C. stereotaxis
   D. thalamotomy
   E. hypophysectomy

617. Cranioplasty may be accomplished with
   A. metallic prosthesis
   B. methyl methacrylate
   C. cerebral revascularization
   D. autogenous bone graft
   E. mersilene mesh

618. Hypophysectomy
   A. is performed for removal of pituitary tumors
   B. explores the floor of the sella turcica through the sphenoid sinus
   C. is a palliative procedure to relieve symptoms of metastatic carcinoma
   D. may use muscle or fat to pack the sella turcica
   E. all of the above

619. Measures to relieve hydrocephalus include
   A. cranioplasty
   B. rhizotomy
   C. ventriculoperitoneal shunt
   D. ventriculoarterial shunt
   E. application of scalp clips

26. PEDIATRIC SURGERY

DIRECTIONS: Each of the questions or incomplete statements below is followed by five suggested answers or completions. Select the most appropriate answer(s).

---

620. A frequently encountered procedure in pediatric surgery is
   A. Keller procedure
   •B. repair of imperforated anus
   •C. repair of esophageal atresia
   •D. resection and pull-through for Hirschsprung's disease
   E. all of the above

621. Hypertrophic pyloric stenosis is a common condition in infants requiring surgery. This
   A. is believed to have a heredity factor involved
   B. is more common in boys
   C. usually is caused by a form of muscular hypertrophy
   D. causes dehydration in the infant
   •E. all of the above

622. Omphalocele repair is replacement of the viscera in the abdominal cavity and reconstruction of the abdominal wall in the newborn. The surgical procedure may consist of
   •A. insertion of silastic sheeting over the sac
   •B. painting the sac and surrounding tissues with 2% mercurochrome to form eschar
   •C. treating the sac with 0.5% silver nitrate
   D. gastrostomy
   E. none of the above

623. Neurogenic bladder is relatively common in infants. This is treated surgically by
   A. reconstruction of the bladder
   •B. diversion of the ureters
   •C. construction of an ileal conduit
   D. repeated dilation of the urethra
   E. none of the above

624. Surgical treatment for aortic stenosis is
   •A. done usually with cardiopulmonary bypass
   B. considered a great risk
   •C. usually a procedure with small risk
   •D. performed through a median sternotomy
   E. none of the above

625. Warm solutions, warm blankets, telethermometer, and hyperthermia mattress used in pediatric surgery are all measures to control
   A. dehydration
   •B. heat loss
   C. infection
   D. cardiopulmonary response
   E. pain

626. The most commonly performed pediatric operation to prevent phimosis is
   A. pyeloureteroplasty
   B. cystoscopy
   C. reconstruction of external genitalia
   •D. circumcision
   E. cryptorchism

627. Surgery for undescended testicles is
   •A. done usually at age 5 or 6
   •B. orchiopexy
   •C. often a two-stage procedure
   D. performed on the infant
   E. an emergency procedure

628. Repair of atresia of the esophagus would include
   •A. right thoracotomy
   B. rib resection
   C. pleural separation
   •D. end-to-end anastomosis
   E. all of the above

629. Excision of aganglionic bowel and reanastomosis to the anus including multiple biopsies and frozen sections to identify normal ganglia is a procedure for
   A. intussusception
   B. Hirschsprung's disease
   C. volvulus
   D. Meckel's diverticulum
   E. none of the above

630. Congenital anomalies that cause obstruction of the colon require a temporary colostomy. These include
   A. Hirschsprung's disease
   B. imperforate anus
   C. atresia
   D. volvulus
   E. all of the above

631. Intussusception may be caused by Meckel's diverticulum, polyps, or hematoma of the bowel. Treatment may be
   A. reduction by barium enema
   B. laparotomy and manual manipulation
   C. resection and pull-through
   D. creation of an intestinal stoma
   E. gastrostomy

632. Wilm's tumor involves the
   A. bowel
   B. stomach
   C. kidney
   D. esophagus
   E. liver

633. A procedure that may be performed in an outpatient clinic or surgicenter is myringotomy with tube insertion. This involves
   A. removal of polyps
   B. making a slit incision in the eardrum
   C. instilling medication
   D. inserting a drainage tube
   E. all of the above

634. Which of the following pediatric surgical procedures would be acceptable for ambulatory or day surgery?
A. Cystoscopy
B. Eye muscle procedures
C. Open reduction of fractures
D. Closed reduction of fractures
E. None of the above

635. Surgical procedures to correct congenital cardiovascular anomalies include
A. repair of atrial septal defect
B. correction of tetralogy of Fallot
C. closure of patent ductus
D. pericardectomy
E. pacemaker insertion

636. Surgical correction of craniosynostosis is
A. ventriculoperitoneal shunt
B. craniectomy
C. correction of spina bifida
D. closure of dural defect
E. none of the above

637. If diagnosed early in infancy, closed reduction with immobilization may correct which congenital deformity?
A. Scoliosis
B. Congenital dislocated hip
C. Tendon deformity
D. Clubfoot
E. Leg length discrepancies

27. CLASSIFICATION, COMPLICATIONS, AND TREATMENT OF BURNS

DIRECTIONS: Each of the questions or incomplete statements below is followed by five suggested answers or completions. Select the most appropriate answer(s).

---

638. The classification of burns by cause includes which of the following?
   A. Electricity
   B. Thermal agents
   C. Chemical agents
   D. Radioactive agents
   •E. All of the above

639. A first degree burn is
   A. caused by mild heat source
   B. reddened
   C. moderately painful
   D. found on intact skin
   •E. all of the above

640. Burns are also classified by degree of damage. There are first degree, second degree, and third degree burns. Characteristics of a third degree burn would be
   A. markedly reddened
   B. severely painful
   •C. appearance is pearly white or charred
   •D. relatively painless
   E. none of the above

641. Classification by extent is known as the rule of nines. Some examples of this would be
   A. the head, neck, and face equal 18%
   B. each upper extremity equals 9%
   C. the anterior surface of the trunk equals 9%
   D. each lower extremity equals 18%
   E. the posterior surface of the trunk equals 18%

642. Regarding the Lund and Brower chart
   A. it considers age a factor in estimating the percentage of body surface burned
   B. percentage sizes differ in infancy and childhood
   C. it is useful in burn assessment
   D. it assists in determining the type of burn therapy
   E. all of the above

643. Initial care of the burn patient includes
   A. stopping the burn process
   B. ensuring a patent airway and instituting IV therapy
   C. massive degloving excision
   D. escharotomy
   E. insertion of Foley catheter

644. Surgical treatment of burn patients may include
   A. covering a partial thickness injury with pigskin
   B. spraying the wound with a type of plastic skin
   C. grafting with skin harvested from cadavers
   D. application of split-thickness sheet graft
   E. all of the above

645. Considerations for patients with extensive burns may include
   A. transfer on a Stryker frame or circo-electric bed
   B. laminar airflow
   C. reverse isolation techniques
   D. plastic isolator
   E. all of the above

646. Serial biopsy cultures
   A. help determine antibiotic or chemotherapeutic agents to be used
   B. monitor growth of microorganisms in the wound
   C. are a form of debridement
   D. promote healing
   E. determine readiness for skin graft

647. Biological dressings applied in the OR may be
- A. meshgrafts
- B. amniotic membranes
- C. heterograft of porcine skin
- D. sulfadiazine cream
- E. heterograft from a living or cadaver donor

28. RADIATION THERAPY

DIRECTIONS: Each of the questions or incomplete statements below is followed by five suggested answers or completions. Select the most appropriate answer(s).

---

648. Radioactive substances are composed of elements which are composed of
    A. gamma rays
    .B. atoms
    C. electrons
    D. roentgens
    E. none of the above

649. An atom which has been made unstable is
    A. an axon
    B. an ion
    •C. an isotope
    .D. radioactive
    E. none of the above

650. Cancer cells are cells
    A. in an active, uncontrolled state of mitosis ("gone wild")
    B. that divide and multiply at an alarming rate of speed
    C. which invade surrounding tissues
    D. which migrate to other parts of the body and become metastatic lesions
    .E. all of the above

651. Radiation therapy used to treat patients is in many forms, such as
    A. x-ray
    B. cobalt 60
    C. radium
    D. radioactive gold isotope
    • E. all of the above

652. Important considerations for patients who have received radiation therapy are
   A. skin should not be prepared and draped
   •B. wound closure may be difficult
   •C. skin in the irradiated area may be fragile and sensitive
   •D. healing may be prolonged
   E. incisional hernias are common

653. Which of the following is not true of radium substitutes (iridium 192, cesium 137, cobalt 60)?
   A. They only remain radioactive for a few years
   •B. They are as hazardous as radium
   C. Afterloading techniques reduce hazards
   D. Radioactive sources do not have to be inserted in the OR
   E. Safety regulations for the use of radium and radium substitutes should be reviewed regularly

654. Primary factors for safe handling of radiation sources include
   A. monitoring devices
   •B. time
   C. assignment rotation
   •D. distance
   •E. shielding

VI

MISCELLANEOUS

29. MISCELLANEOUS

DIRECTIONS: Each of the questions or incomplete statements below is followed by five suggested answers or completions. Select the most appropriate answer(s).

---

655. A Wertheim procedure is
   - •A. a radical abdominal hysterectomy
   - •B. removal of uterus, tubes, ovaries, proximal vagina, bilateral lymph nodes
   - C. the same as a Marshall-Marchetti procedure
   - D. the removal of the bladder and the creation of an ileal loop
   - E. usually a procedure performed only on men, resection of spermatic cord

656. An infant between the ages of 4 and 6 weeks is diagnosed as having hypertrophied stenosis of the pyloric sphincter. What procedure corrects this?
   - A. There is no procedure to correct it; it will resolve itself once solid food is taken
   - •B. Ramstedt-Fredet procedure
   - C. Dwyer procedure
   - D. Billroth II
   - E. Harrington technique

657. Marlex mesh
   - A. is used for cardiovascular procedures, particularly open heart surgery
   - •B. is used for additional strength and repair of inguinal or incisional hernias
   - •C. may be used to repair thoracic wall defects
   - •D. after 6 weeks forms a strong fibrous wall; fibrous tissue easily grows through mesh
   - E. all of the above

658. What is a sump drain?
 · A. A plastic or rubber catheter that is attached to suction
 B. A urinary drainage tube
 C. A thoracic drainage tube
 D. A larger version of a Jackson-Pratt drain
 E. A special drain used for hydrocephalics

659. The bovine heterograft
 · A. is composed of a specially selected bovine carotid artery
 · B. serves as a substitute passageway for blood
 · C. is intended to be used as a segmental arterial replacement, arterial bypass or shunt, or arterial patch graft
 D. creates a direct arteriovenous fistula between the radial artery and the cephalic vein
 E. none of the above

660. Regarding surgical treatment of children with exstrophy of the bladder
 A. this is a congenital deformity in which there is open bladder herniation
 B. it requires reconstruction of the lower abdominal wall and external genitalia
 C. it must make a pathway for urination
 D. it would require the expertise of a urologist
 · E. all of the above

661. Advantages of stapling instruments include which of the following?
 A. Reduced possibility of infection and tissue reaction
 B. Stapled tissues undergo less trauma
 C. Reduced operating time
 · D. All of the above
 E. None of the above

662. If a procedure is done under local anesthesia, the surgeon may choose to use Xylocaine 1% with epinephrine. What is the purpose of the epinephrine?
 A. Reduces bleeding at the operative site because it is a vasoconstrictor
 B. Prolongs effects of Xylocaine
 C. Allows for smaller quantities of Xylocaine to be used
 · D. All of the above
 E. A only

663. What instruments would be included in the set-up for mandibular or maxillary osteotomies?
   A. Assorted sizes of wire, wire cutters
   B. Hand drill or air drill 100 with assorted burrs
   C. Mouth gag, tonsil suction, Frazier suction, tongue retractor
   D. Osteotomes, periosteal elevators, ribbon retractors
   E. All of the above

664. What are some complications of laparoscopy?
   A. The only complication reported is that of bowel perforation
   B. Hemorrhage or piercing of major abdominal vessel
   C. Gastritis
   D. Embolism, because of IV CO_2 injection
   E. All of the above

665. Cryosurgery is performed
   A. by use of a special instrument
   B. by quick cooling action to very low temperatures
   C. only in ophthalmic procedures
   D. by use of liquid nitrogen, CO_2, or freon
   E. all of the above

666. What vitamin is essential for blood clotting?
   A. Vitamin C
   B. Vitamin K
   C. Vitamin B_1
   D. Vitamin E
   E. Vitamin B_{12}

667. What is abdominoplasty?
   A. Removal of adipose tissue from abdomen
   B. Removal of diseased sinus membrane
   C. Removal of pancreas
   D. Removal of diseased bone marrow
   E. None of the above

668. Outpatient surgery facilities are increasing in numbers. Reasons for this are
   A. the escalating costs of inpatient hospital care
   B. better utilization of hospital facilities
   C. the ability to integrate this service into major OR facilities
   D. a recovery room is not required
   E. it requires less concern for the design of the facility

669. Which of the following are true regarding outpatients or patients having one-day surgery?
   A. They may or may not be administered general anesthesia
   B. Some independent facilities provide overnight rooms
   C. Conduct of OR personnel requires special considerations for the outpatient
   D. Outpatients usually require fewer lab tests
   •E. All of the above

670. Charnley, Charnley-Mueller, Bechtol, and Aufranc-Turner are names of
   A. retractors used in hip surgery
   B. names of surgical orthopedic procedures
   C. orthopedic drills
   •D. hip prostheses
   E. none of the above

671. Pancreatic transplants
   A. have never been done on humans
   •B. are being investigated because of the failure of exogenous insulin to halt diabetic complications
   •C. were first done in 1966
   •D. have been carried out in a small number of patients
   E. all of the above

672. Liver transplants are complicated procedures because of which of the following?
   A. Multiple arterial anastomoses
   B. Biliary duct anastomosis
   C. Derangements in the coagulation mechanism
   D. Metabolic complications
   •E. All of the above

673. Which of the following are considered factors having a direct relationship to the incidence of wound infection?
   A. Short preoperative hospitalization
   B. Preoperative bathing
   •C. Long surgical procedures
   D. Shaving less than 2 hr before surgery
   •E. Use of electrosurgical knife

674. Ultrasonography
   - A. is automated and does not require great skill of the operator
   - B. is less costly than CT scans
   - C. involves radiation exposure
   - D. can demonstrate pancreatic cysts and pseudocysts
   - E. can demonstrate cystic or solid nature of ovarian masses

675. Which of the following are true of penile implants?
   - A. Have a low success rate of ending impotence
   - B. May be inflatable
   - C. May be semirigid
   - D. Mechanical complication is common with the semi-rigid prosthesis
   - E. Surgical procedure for insertion of the inflatable prosthesis is less complicated than the semirigid

676. Bone marrow harvest requires that the patient usually be placed in what position?
   - A. Lithotomy
   - B. Fowler's
   - C. Prone
   - D. Supine
   - E. Left lateral

677. Nissen fundoplication
   - A. prevents esophageal reflux
   - B. is usually done through an upper median laparotomy
   - C. requires placement of a large lumen gastric tube
   - D. is repair of hiatus hernia
   - E. all of the above

678. The Broviac catheter is
   - A. for long-term use, indwelling
   - B. used for dialysis
   - C. used to administer IV fluids, chemotherapy, antibiotics, and hyperalimentation
   - D. is inserted into the femoral vein
   - E. is a urology catheter

679. Correction of scoliosis and other severe spinal deformities may include which of the following instrumentation?
• A. Harrington system
• B. Dwyer spinal instrumentation
• C. Plaster body cast
D. Moore's prosthesis
E. All of the above

680. In the event of cardiac arrest, what are the most important initial elements of resuscitation?
• A. Patent airway
• B. Artificial ventilation
• C. External cardiac compression
D. Precordial thump
E. All of the above

681. Chest injuries may result in a loss of negative pressure within the pleural cavity. What are priorities in this emergency situation?
• A. Ensure airway
B. Secure portable x-rays
• C. Assist with physical exam and insertion of chest tube
• D. Elevate head and chest unless the patient is in shock
E. None of the above

682. Emergency management of craniocerebral injuries include which of the following?
A. Keep patient in semisitting position
• B. Maintain airway
• C. Assess level of responsiveness
• D. Assist with physical exam and control of hemorrhage and shock
E. All of the above

683. Which would NOT be a biophysical test of fetal status?
A. Ultrasound
B. Amniography or amnioscopy
C. Fetoscopy
• D. Epidural block
E. Electronic fetal monitoring

684. Which of the following could be causes of fetal distress?
A. Umbilical cord problems
B. Prematurity
C. Maternal hypotension
D. Intrauterine growth retardation
• E. All of the above

685. Which of the following is premature separation of the placenta from the wall of the uterus?
   A. Placenta previa
   B. Uterine atony
   •C. Abruptio placenta
   D. Lacerated perineum
   E. Third-stage hemorrhage

686. Guidelines for taking vital signs include which of the following?
   •A. Record immediately
   •B. Seek assistance if difficult to read or take
   •C. Alert nurse or physician if abnormal
   D. Never repeat
   E. All of the above

687. Regarding chest tubes left in place to drain the thoracic cavity
   •A. they may be attached to an underwater seal drainage system
   •B. they are placed to drain fluid and air from the chest cavity
   C. they need not be clamped when disconnected
   D. they can be in any position in relation to the drainage system
   E. drainage system need not be sterile

688. Catheterization of the bladder requires
   A. proper patient positioning
   B. strict aseptic technique
   C. testing of the catheter balloon before insertion
   D. catheter lubrication
   •E. all of the above

689. Invasive monitoring techniques include
   A. ECG
   •B. CVP
   C. Doppler
   •D. arterial
   •E. pulmonary artery pressure

690. Which of the following are true of electrocautery?
- . A. Proper ground is necessary to complete a safe electrical circuit
- • B. Solid-state models allow for pinpoint cautery
- C. Continued increase in power is acceptable if desired results not obtained
- . D. It uses a high-frequency electrical force to cauterize bleeding vessels
- E. All of the above

691. Which of the following are NOT true of tourniquets?
- . A. They totally prevent arterial flow
- B. Area where applied must be padded with cotton
- C. Gauge must be checked for accuracy and proper working order
- D. Surgeon should be notified of length of tourniquet time at regular intervals
- E. Use of tourniquet allows clear view of the operative site

ANSWERS AND COMMENTS

The authors have made every effort to thoroughly verify the answers to the questions which appear on the preceding pages. However, as in any text, some inaccuracies and ambiguities may occur; therefore, if in doubt, please consult your references.

The Publisher

I. Introduction

1. (E) Temperature should be controlled between 68-75° F and humidity at a minimum of 50% to aid in the control of static electricity. High-flow unidirectional ventilation systems provide a cleaner OR environment and may reduce the potential for infection. There should be up to 25 room air exchanges per hour. REF. 20, pp. 25-26

2. (B) Trans is a prefix meaning through, across, or beyond, i.e., transfusion. REF. 43, p. 7

3. (D) Itis is a suffix meaning inflammation of, i.e., tonsillitis. REF. 43, p. 10

4. (A) An infarct is an area of necrosis following cessation of blood supply, i.e., mesenteric infarct. REF. 43, p. 12

5. (C) Ectomy is a suffix meaning surgical excision of, i.e., appendectomy. REF. 43, p. 9

6. (D) Ostomy is the creation of a new artificial opening, i.e., colostomy. REF. 43, p. 10

7. (C) Ischemia is a deficiency of blood in a body part. REF. 11, p. 288

8. (C) Abduction is a movement whereby a body part is drawn away from the main axis or the axis of a limb. REF. 42, p. 607

9. (B,C) The purpose of both these institutions is to: (1) establish standards for the operation of hospitals; and (2) evaluate whether a hospital meets those standards. REF. 18, p. 1275

II. Basic Sciences

10. (D) Dividing the body by a horizontal cut into upper and lower portions gives a transverse section. REF. 11, p. 2

11. (A) Metabolism is the chemical transformation that takes place in the body, the release of energy, and the excretion of waste. REF. 42, p. 355

12. (E) Connective tissue is classified according to the type and density of its fibers and its cellular organization. Bone, cartilage, adipose, and areolar are just a few examples of connective tissue. REF. 11, pp. 8-11

13. (D) Articulation is the way in which joints are arranged. REF. 42, p. 103

14. (B) Arthritis is the inflammation of a joint. REF. 42, p. 608

15. (B) The occipital bone is located at the posterior position of the skull. REF. 20, p. 701

16. (A,B) The skeletal muscles that execute movement by will are striated and are known as voluntary. REF. 11, p. 57

17. (B) The cavity and capsule of the synovial joint is lined with a synovial membrane, which elaborates a clear fluid resembling egg albumin. This synovial fluid lubricates the joint and nourishes the cartilage. REF. 11, pp. 52-53

18. (B) Metacarpophalangeal is a synovial joint with biaxial movement. Interphalangeal is also a synovial joint but with uniaxial movement. REF. 11, p. 853

19. (A,D) There are common types of movement that occur especially in limb joints, flexion or bending and its opposite, extension or straightening. REF. 11, p. 53

20. (B) Protraction is the protrusion outward of some body part, i. e. , lower jaw. REF. 42, p. 84

21. (C) The elbow represents a joint between the humerus (upper arm) and ulna and radius (lower arm). REF. 42, p. 87

22. (C) The diaphysis is the main shaft found in long bones, i. e. , femur, humerus. REF. 42, p. 89

23. (B) Ossification begins when bone-forming cells or osteoblasts appear in the body. These cells secrete or form the organic intercellular substance of bone. REF. 11, p. 31

24. (A,D) Osteoporosis is a weakening of the skeleton due to loss of minerals and excessive osteoclast activity. The cause is variable but linked to decreased normal activity in postmenopausal women. REF. 42, p. 100

25. (B) Tendons are composed of parallel fibers of collagen so strong that under severe stress it is not uncommon for the bony attachment of tendon to tear away from the bone itself rather than for the tendon to break. REF. 42, p. 102

26. (A,B,C) Cartilage consists of hyaline, elastic fibrous, and inelastic fibrous varieties. Usually surrounded by a perichondrium, cartilage contains much more glycoprotein-ground substance than collagen. REF. 42, p. 108

27. (A) A typical bone is surrounded by a periosteal membrane and possesses an outer crust of compact bone and an inner filling of cancellous bone and marrow.

28. (E) Several types of arthritic disorders occur: infectious, gouty, osteoid, and rheumatoid. REF. 42, p. 106

29. (E) The purpose of immobilization is to hold bone fragments in contact with each other until healing takes place. Immobilization restricts movement of the injured part and provides protection. REF. 19, pp. 854-855

30. (E) Internal fixation is achieved by using a metal device. There are a wide variety of metal pins, wires, intramedullary rods, compression plates, and nails available for internal stabilization. REF. 19, p. 864

31. (B,C) The halo cast is an apparatus used to immobilize the cervical spine following a cervical spine fusion or fracture. REF. 19, p. 864

32. (C) Deep fascia is the tough, fibrous tissue covering muscles, blood vessels, and nerves. REF. 11, p. 15

33. (A) A cluster of nerve cell bodies outside the central nervous system is referred to as a ganglion. REF. 11, p. 82

34. (A) The outermost layer is called the dura mater. The most superficial part is the periosteal dura, which is actually the periosteum or inner covering of the cranial bones. REF. 11, p. 90

35. (B) The pia mater is the innermost layer of meninges; it is delicate and transparent, follows the contours of the brain, and is adherent to it. REF. 11, p. 90

36. (B) The cerebrospinal fluid circulates through the ventricles of the brain, escapes through the three openings in the fourth ventricle, and continues into the subarachnoid space around the brain and spinal cord. REF. 11, p. 91

37. (A) The largest part of the human brain is the cerebrum, which contains the highest centers of the nervous system. REF. 11, p. 103

38. (A, B) The spinal cord has two main functions: (1) to serve as a reflex center; and (2) to serve as a pathway for conducting impulses either to or from higher parts of the neuraxis. REF. 11, p. 96

39. (D) The brain gives rise to twelve pairs of cranial nerves, which are unlike the spinal nerves. Three pairs are purely sensory, whereas the other nine contain both sensory and motor fibers. REF. 11, p. 111

40. (A,D) The two principal divisions of the nervous system are the central nervous system (CNS) and the peripheral nervous system (PNS). The CNS consists of the brain and spinal cord. The PNS is made up of the sensory receptors and the nerves, which are the communication lines. REF. 42, p. 207

41. (A,D) The PNS is subdivided into somatic and autonomic portions. Both systems have sensory nerves (afferent) and motor nerves (efferent). REF. 42, p. 209

42. (A,B) In general, the sympathetic nerves operate to stimulate organs and to mobilize energy, especially in response to stress. REF. 42, p. 209

43. (B) Dendrites are typically short, highly branched fibers specialized to receive neural impulses. REF. 42, p. 212

44. (E) In multiple sclerosis, which is a neurological disease, patches of myelin deteriorate at irregular intervals along the length of neurons and are replaced by scar tissue. REF. 42, p. 213

45. (E) The simplest example of a neural response in human beings is the reflex action, which is a predictable automatic response to a specific stimulus. REF. 42, p. 216

46. (B) Nerves from the lower region of the cord run caudally to below the level of the conus medullaris before they leave the vertebral canal. Because of their resemblance to a horse's tail, they are aptly known as the cauda equina. REF. 42, p. 233

47. (A,C,D) From the outside inward the meninges are called the dura mater, arachnoid, and pia mater. REF. 42, p. 233

48. (A,B) The spinal cord has two main functions: (1) it controls many reflex activities of the body; and (2) it transmits information back and forth to the brain via its ascending and descending tracts. REF. 42, pp. 236-237

49. (E) The hypothalamus has a hand in regulating many mechanisms essential to maintaining homeostasis. REF. 42, pp. 242-243

50. (C) The cerebrum is partially divided into right and left cerebral hemispheres. Each hemisphere is divided into six lobes: frontal, parietal, occipital, temporal, central, and limbic. REF. 42, p. 244

51. (C) The most anterior portion of each frontal lobe is known as the prefrontal lobe. REF. 42, p. 247

52. (A) Parkinson's disease is a disorder in which movement is shaky and difficult. Some say that the transmitter substance, dopamine, does not play an important role in motor function. REF. 42, p. 249

53. (D) There are twelve pairs of cranial nerves which emerge from the brain itself. REF. 42, p. 259

54. (A) There are thirty-one pairs of spinal nerves which emerge from the spinal cord. Eight pairs of cervical, twelve pairs of thoracic, five pairs of lumbar, five pairs of sacral, and one pair of coccygeal. REF. 42, p. 261

55. (C) Food is taken into the body, chewed and swallowed, and both mechanically and chemically broken down. Once broken down or digested, it is then small enough to pass through the wall of the gastrointestinal (GI) tract and into the blood or lymph (the process of absorption). Undigested and unabsorbed food is eliminated from the body by the process of defecation. REF. 42, p. 317

56. (B) The mucous membranes of the mouth contain several small glands that produce a secretion called saliva. In addition, there are three pairs of larger salivary glands that are not located in the mouth cavity but discharge saliva into it. They are known as the parotid, submandibular, and sublingual glands. REF. 11, p. 189

57. (E) The pharynx is common to both the respiratory and digestive systems. REF. 11, p. 165

58. (A) The esophagus (gullet) is a collapsible tube 10 in. long lying posterior to the trachea. REF. 11, p. 187

59. (E) The stomach lies in the upper part of the abdominal cavity, just below the diaphragm. The opening between the esophagus and the stomach is the cardiac orifice. REF. 11, p. 189

60. (B) The fundus is that portion of the stomach lying above a line drawn through the cardiac orifice. REF. 11, p. 190

61. (A) The first 12 in. of the small intestine is the duodenum. The jejunum forms the next two-fifths (about 8 ft) of the small intestine. The ileum forms the distal portion of the tube and is about 12 ft long. REF. 11, p. 191

62. (A) The most distal portion of the stomach is known as the pylorus. REF. 11, p. 190

63. (A) In the small intestine, the process of absorption occurs. This refers to the passage of prepared material (food) from the digestive tract to the blood. From there the absorbed material is utilized by the body cells by the process of metabolism. REF. 11, p. 123

64. (E) The large intestine extends from the small intestine at the ileocecal orifice to the ascending, the transverse, the descending, the sigmoid, the rectum, and continues to the anus. REF. 11, pp. 192-193

65. (D) The pancreas is a fixed structure lying transversely behind the stomach in the upper abdomen. The head of the pancreas is fixed to the curve of the duodenum and shares the same blood supply. REF. 20, p. 182

66. (C) The ampulla (or papilla) of Vater is formed by the dilated junction of the two ducts, pancreatic (duct of Wirsung) and the common bile duct. REF. 5, p. 182.

67. (A) The pancreas contains a group of cells called islets or islands of Langerhans, which secrete hormones into the blood capillaries. These hormones are called insulin and glucagon. REF. 5, p. 182

68. (A) The common hepatic duct merges with the cystic duct from the gallbladder to form the common bile duct. REF. 5, p. 182

69. (B) The gallbladder lies in the sulcus of the undersurface of the right lobe of the liver and terminates in the cystic duct. The digestive system provides a channel for the flow of bile to the gallbladder, where it becomes highly concentrated during the storage period. REF. 5, p. 8

70. (B) Hemolysis is a chemical term in which there is premature red blood cell destruction, whether due to reduction in red cell lite or to random cell destruction. REF. 5, p. 174

71. (B) The hematocrit is a measure of the volume of red cells per unit volume of blood. The hematocrit of circulating blood varies in different parts of the vascular tree. REF. 5, p. 296

72. (E) The terms leukocyte and white blood cells refer to any of the nucleated cells normally present in blood, the major function of which is defense against foreign invaders. REF. 5, p. 253

73. (E) Platelets or thrombolytes are cell fragments that adhere to injured blood vessels and form hemostatic plugs that help to staunch the flow of blood from damaged blood vessels. REF. 5, p. 401

74. (D) An embolism may be a clot particle, foreign body, air, fat, or tumor that circulates through the bloodstream and becomes lodged as the vessel decreases in size. REF. 5, p. 434

75. (B) A low hematocrit indicates deficiency of red blood cells; a high reading may be an indication of polycythemia, too many red cells. REF. 42, p. 385

76. (C) Red blood cells or erythrocytes are the most numerous and one of the most specialized cell types in the body. REF. 4, p. 387

77. (C) Normal adult values: 12-15 g/100 ml for women; 14-17 g/100 ml for men. REF. 4, p. 394

78. (A) Fibrin is an insoluble fibrous protein that reinforces the platelet plug. This reaction is catalyzed by a substance called thrombin. REF. 4, p. 395

79. (C) Platelets number about 300,000/ml of circulating blood. Platelets function to stop bleeding in two ways. They physically plug any break in a blood vessel wall and they release chemicals that promote clotting. REF. 4, p. 395

80. (C) All arteries carry blood away from the heart to the organs and tissues of the body. REF. 4, p. 398

81. (C) In the liver, spleen, and bone marrow, arterioles and venules are connected by passages known as sinusoids, rather than by typical capillaries. REF. 4, p. 399

82. (D) Plasma contains 92% water, 7% protein, a sprinkling of salts, and a vast array of other materials. REF. 42, p. 386

83. (B) In a man weighing about 70 kg (154 lb), the blood volume should be about 5.6 L (6 qt). REF. 42, p. 385

84. (C) The normal circulating blood volume is about 8% of body weight. REF. 42, p. 385

85. (A) The heart, a hollow muscular organ that acts as a power pump for the circulating system, is enclosed in a pericardial sac (pericardium) forming the middle subdivision of the lower part of the mediastinum. REF. 20, p. 379

86. (C) The heart wall is composed of three layers: the epicardium (outermost layer), the myocardium (muscular layer), and the endocardium (inner layer). REF. 20, p. 379

87. (A,B) There are three openings into the right atrium. One is the coronary sinus, which returns venous blood collected from the veins draining the heart muscle itself. The other two are the superior vena cava and the inferior vena cava. These vessels return all venous blood from the organs of the body. REF. 11, p. 140

88. (C) The heart chambers have four valves: two atrioventricular valves and two semilunar valves. The two atrioventricular valves are located between the atrium and ventricle of each side of the heart. The right atrioventricular valve is commonly called the tricuspid valve. REF. 20, p. 379

89. (D) The SA node is the main pacemaker of the heart and is located in the upper right atrium near the superior vena cava. It usually generates 60-100 impulses/min in the adult. REF. 35, p. 914

90. (B) The wave of atrial contraction is picked up by the AV node and spreads to the AV bundle. From here, via the bundle branches and fibers, the wave of contraction spreads throughout the ventricular walls. REF. 11, p. 142

91. (B) During diastole, the ventricles relax and the atria contract, pumping blood through the atrioventricular valves into the ventricles. REF. 20, p. 379

92. (D) Atrial fibrillation occurs when the sinus node no longer controls the rhythm of the heart and the atria no longer

contract in coordination. In ventricular fibrillation, the coordinated contraction of the ventricles is replaced by rapid, irregular twitching of the ventricular muscles. REF. 35, pp. 1001-1003

93. (A) In sinus tachycardia the heart rate is greater than 100 beats/min. REF. 35, p. 997

94. (C) In sinus bradycardia the heart rate falls below 60 beats/min. REF. 35, p. 997

95. (A,B) Epinephrine and adrenaline are both vasoconstrictors and affect the heart rate by increasing frequency and force. REF. 34, p. 1983

96. (B) The jejunum and ileum are suspended by the mesentery, which is attached to the posterior abdominal wall. The free border of the mesentery contains branches of the superior mesenteric artery. The blood supply to the ascending and transverse colons comes from the superior mesenteric artery, and the blood supply to the descending colon and rectum comes from the inferior mesenteric artery. REF. 20, pp. 206-209

97. (D) The descending aorta bifurcates at the fourth lumbar vertebra into the right and left common iliacs (the right and left internal and external iliac) to the right and left femorals. REF. 11, p. 411

98. (C) The circle of Willis is located at the base of the brain. The circle of Willis is a ring of blood vessels around the stalk of the pituitary gland and the optic chiasma. REF. 20, p. 707

99. (A, B, C) The arterial blood supply to the liver is maintained by the hepatic artery. Venous blood from the stomach, intestines, spleen, and pancreas is carried to the liver by the portal vein and its branches. REF. 20, p. 182

100. (E) The heart is equipped with its own complex of blood vessels, known as the coronary circulation. The coronary circulation consists of the left and right coronary arteries and the circumflex and posterior descending branches. REF. 42, p. 403

101. (A,B,D) The visceral and parietal branches of the thoracic aorta supply oxygenated blood to the bronchi of lungs, esophagus, intercostals, and other chest muscles. REF. 42, p. 405

102. (A) Umbrella filters are used to create partial occlusion of the inferior vena cava to prevent pulmonary embolisms. REF. 35, pp. 442-443

103. (C) The liver is supplied with oxygenated blood by the hepatic arteries. Its branches feed into the hepatic sinuses, where its blood mixes with the venous blood from the hepatic portal vein. REF. 42, p. 416

104. (E) In summary, blood flows through the vessels to the pulmonary circulation in the following sequence: right atrium to right ventricle to pulmonary trunk to pulmonary artery to pulmonary arterioles to pulmonary capillaries to pulmonary venules to pulmonary veins to left atrium. REF. 42, p. 403

105. (A,B,C) Blood is supplied to the esophagus from branches of the inferior thyroid, thoracic aorta, and celiac arteries. REF. 20, p. 206

106. (A) The blood supply to the ascending colon, hepatic flexure, and transverse colon comes from the superior mesenteric artery, whereas the blood supply to the descending colon and rectum comes from the inferior mesenteric artery. REF. 20, p. 209

107. (B) The blood supply of the kidney is conveyed through the renal artery, a large branch of the aorta, and leaves the kidney through the renal vein. REF. 20, p. 236

108. (A,B) Each tube receives its blood supply from the branches of the uterine and ovarian arteries. REF. 20, p. 308

109. (E) On the medial side of each kidney is a concave area known as the hilum through which the renal artery and vein enter and leave. REF. 20, p. 236

110. (A) <u>Pyelo</u> refers to the kidney pelvis.

111. (B) Microscopic examination of the kidney reveals that it is composed of perhaps a million or more microscopic units called nephrons, plus the collecting ducts that gather the product of these nephrons. REF. 42, p. 495

112. (D) Normal urine is a clear, amber-colored liquid. In certain diseases the urine will contain substances not normally found, i.e., the presence of blood (hematuria), sugar (glycosuria), or pus (pyuria). REF. 11, p. 224

113. (B) The renal pelvis is a funnel-shaped structure. It lies posterior to the renal vascular pedicle and divides into several branches within the kidney called calyces. REF. 20, p. 236

114. (A) The urinary meatus opens anterior to the opening of the vagina. REF. 11, p. 226

115. (C) Arteries, veins, nerves, and conducting tubes are structures which are encased by the cremaster muscle and by layers of fascia which constitute the spermatic cord. REF. 42, p. 546

116. (C) The prostate gland lies under the urinary bladder, its base adjoining the inferior aspect of the bladder. REF. 11, p. 263

117. (A, B, C) The accessory reproductive glands include the seminal vesicle, prostate gland, and bulbourethral gland. The seminal vesicle unites with the vas deferens and produces protein and fructose for sperm cell nutrition. REF. 20, p. 238

118. (B) On the medial side of each kidney is a concave area known as the hilum through which the renal artery and vein enter and leave. REF. 42, p. 493

119. (B) The permeability of the collecting ducts to water varies under the control of ADH, which is secreted by the posterior pituitary gland. REF. 42, p. 503

120. (C) Polyuria occurs most often in diabetes insipidus. It is characterized by an increased urine output which is chronically dilute. REF. 42, p. 503

121. (A, B, C) There are several disease conditions which cause renal failure: pyelonephritis (kidney infection), glomerulonephritis, and actite tubular necrosis. REF. 42, pp. 506-507

122. (E) Gout is defective excretion of blood uric acid. The disease is extremely painful due to the deposits of uric acid crystals commonly found in the joint cavities. REF. 42, p. 507

123. (C) Only the liver compares to the kidney in its ability to adjust and maintain a healthy environment for the cells of the body. REF. 42, p. 509

124. (C) Micturition is the ability of the bladder to empty itself of urine when necessary. REF. 42, p. 509

125. (C) The urinary bladder consist of three layers: the inner transitional epithelium, the middle cross-grained detrusor muscle, and the outer serosa. REF. 42, p. 510

126. (A) The ureters deliver urine into the bladder by a periodic wavelike motion known as peristalsis. REF. 42, p. 510

127. (C) The perineum is an almond-shaped area bounded posteriorly by the tip of the coccyx and anteriorly by the symphysis pelvis. REF. 11, p. 272

128. (A, B, C) The ovaries are homologous with the testes of the male. They produce ova after puberty. The hormone estrogen is secreted by the ovarian follicle and the hormone progesterone is secreted by the corpus luteum. REF. 20, p. 308

129. (A) An ectopic pregnancy is one in which the fertilized ovum becomes embedded outside the body of the uterus. Since it is almost always located in the fallopian tube, the term tubal pregnancy is often used. REF. 35, p. 1422

130. (D) The uterus, which occupies a central place in the pelvis, is a pecan-shaped organ situated between the bladder and the rectum. REF. 20, p. 305

131. (C) The uterus lies posterior to the bladder and anterior to the rectum. The uterine body has three layers: (1) the

outer peritoneal or serous layer; (2) the myometrium or muscular layer; and (3) the endometrium or muscosal layer. REF. 20, p. 308

132. (A) The root word for breast is <u>mast</u>. REF. 11, p. 294

133. (C,D) The paired ovaries (female gonads) produce ova, estrogen, and progesterone. REF. 42, p. 551

134. (B) The fimbriae are long, fingerlike projections. REF. 42, p. 554

135. (B,C) Inflammation of the uterine tubes is most often caused by gonorrheal infection. The scarring which sometimes results may partially constrict the tube and cause sterility. REF. 42, p. 555

136. (B) A tipped uterus is one that has shifted from the normal position. Normally the uterus is flexed so that it makes a right angle with the vagina. REF. 42, p. 555

137. (B) Laparoscopy provides visualization of the pelvic organs as is seen when a diagnostic laparotomy is performed. REF. 20, p. 333

138. (C) The epiglottis is a slightly curled leaf-shaped, elastic fibrous membrane. When the cricothyroid muscle constricts, it pulls the thyroid cartilage and the cricoid cartilage, thereby tightening the vocal cords and closing the glottis. REF. 20, p. 630

139. (C) There are two pleural membranes: the parietal pleura, which lines the inner surface of the thorax, and the visceral pleura, which is a serous secretion existing between these two membranes acting as a lubricant to minimize friction. REF. 20, p. 348

140. (E) Upon visualization of the mediastinium via direct vision through a mediastinoscope, you can see the heart, lymph nodes, vessels, tracheobronchial junction, and esophagus. REF. 20, p. 348

141. (A,C) During inspiration the external intercostals lift the ribs up and out. At the same time, the diaphragm contracts, enlarging the chest cavity from the bottom. This double action sucks air into the lungs. REF. 42, p. 480

142. (A) In the medulla of the brain there is a collection of neurons sometimes called the respiratory pacemaker. It governs both inspiration and expiration. REF. 42, p. 481

143. (B) Dyspnea is defined as labored or difficult breathing. REF. 11, p. 172

144. (C) Apnea is defined as the cessation of breathing. REF. 11, p. 172

145. (A) Hypoxia is a deficiency of oxygen to the body. Anoxia is absence of oxygen to the body. REF. 11, p. 178

146. (A, B, C) Chest tubes provide a conduit for drainage of blood and other fluid from the intrapleural or mediastinal space. They also provide for reestablishment of a negative pressure in the intrapleural space. REF. 20, p. 356

147. (A, B, C) Bronchoscopy, esophagoscopy, and mediastinoscopy are pertinent to thoracic surgery and are used as diagnostic and therapeutic procedures. REF. 20, pp. 370-372

148. (E) Lung biopsy is resection of a small portion of the lung for diagnosis. Segmental resection is removal of individual branch or vascular segments of the pulmonary lobe. Wedge resection is excision of a small wedge-shaped section of the lobe. Lobectomy is the excision of one or more lobes of the lung. REF. 20, pp. 370-372

149. (B) A liberal application of sterile talcum powder to the visceral and parietal pleural surfaces stimulates the growth of adhesion between the pleurae. The creation of pleural adhesion is indicated in the presence of recurrent idiopathic spontaneous pneumothorax. REF. 20, p. 375

150. (B) Pneumonectomy is performed to treat malignant neoplasm of the lung. REF. 20, p. 374

151. (B, C) The eye is really an extension of the brain and is considered a part of the central nervous system. REF. 11, p. 119

152. (A) The moist membranes that cover the white of the eyes and line the upper and lower lids are called the conjunctivas. REF. 42, p. 286

153. (B, C) Tears are secreted by the supraorbital lacrimal glands and accessory conjunctival glands. Tears flow at all times to wash away foreign particles, to lubricate the lids, and to keep the transparent cornea moist. REF. 42, p. 286

154. (A) The sclera is the posterior part of the external tumic. The external protection fibrous tumic is comprised of the cornea and sclera. REF. 42, p. 655

155. (A, B, C) The cornea is the anterior, transparent part of the external tumic and is continuous with the sclera. The cornea serves as a window through which light rays pass to the retina. REF. 42, p. 655

156. (C) The iris is a thin membrane, the anterior portion of the middle tumic, and is situated in front of the lens. The iris regulates the amount of light entering the eye. REF. 42, pp. 655-656

157. (B) The image produced by the lens and cornea lies on the retina, and it is the retina's response to this image that produces the sensations of vision. REF. 42, p. 296

158. (D) Conduction of visual impulses to the cortex is via the two optic nerves that pass posteriorly out of the bony orbits through the optic canals. REF. 11, p. 120

159. (B) The fovea centralis is the area of the keenest vision. It is here that the cones are located; they are responsible for daylight vision. They interpret fine detail, contrast, and color. REF. 11, p. 120

160. (A) When the lens becomes opaque, such as in old age, it is known as a cataract. The treatment for a cataract is surgical removal, combined with strong glasses to compensate for the absence of the lens. REF. 42, p. 295

161. (A, C) Mydriatric drugs dilate the pupil but permit the patient to focus. Cycloplegic drugs dilate the pupil and also prevent focusing of the eye. REF. 20, p. 660

162. (C) Strabismus is the inability to direct the two eyes at the same object because of lack of coordination of the extraoccular muscles. REF. 20, p. 672

163. (B) Keratoplasty is the grafting of corneal tissue from one human eye to another. REF. 20, p. 677

164. (C) Iridectomy is the removal of a section of the iris to reestablish communication between the posterior and anterior chambers. This establishes the outflow of aqueous fluid. It is done to treat actite, subactite, and chronic glaucoma. REF. 20, p. 688

165. (A) The intracapsular method of cataract removal consists of removing the lens within the capsule. In the extracapsular method, the anterior portion of the capsule is first ruptured and removed and the lens cortex and muscleus expressed for eye. REF. 20, p. 682

166. (A, B, C) The endocrine system works closely with the nervous system to maintain the steady state of the body. Endocrine control depends upon chemical messengers called hormones produced by endocrine glands. REF. 42, p. 512

167. (E) Anterior pituitary hormones influence other endocrine glands. Dysfunction of the anterior pituitary gland may cause symptoms of malfunction in other glands, leading to various disease conditions. REF. 35, p. 568

168. (E) Hyperthyroidism, or hyperactivity of the thyroid gland, may be called thyrotoxicosis, toxic goiter, or Graves' disease. The gland becomes enlarged and secretes increased quantities of thyroid hormone. REF. 35, p. 571

169. (B,C,D) Simple goiter or hyperplasia results from impaired thyroid function. Simple goiter can be prevented by eating foods that contain iodine or by using iodized salt. REF. 35, p. 570-571

170. (E) Calcium is needed for blood coagulation; smooth, skeletal, and cardiac muscle function; nerve function; and bone and teeth formation. REF. 35, p. 312

171. (A) The adrenal medulla secretes epinephrine and norepinephrine, which help the body to react to emergency situations. These hormones increase heart rate, metabolic rate, and strength of muscle contraction. REF. 42, p. 534

172. (C) The islets of Langerhans secrete insulin, which decreases blood sugar, and glucagon, which increases blood sugar levels. REF. 42, p. 537

173. (D) Electrolytes are chemical compounds in solution that have the ability to conduct an electrical current. In solution, electrolytes break into charged particles called ions. When positively charged, they are called cations and when negatively charged are called anions. REF. 35

174. (A) The influence of ADH upon the kidney tubule allows water to be reabsorbed in an amount compatible with the maintenance of proper fluid balance. REF. 35, p. 1229

175. (B) Somatotropin is concerned with growth of bones, muscles, cells. It affects metabolism and is an insulin antagonist. REF. 35, p. 538

176. (C) Very small amounts of both androgens (masculine effect) and estrogens (female hormone) are secreted by the adrenal cortex in both sexes. REF. 42, p. 531

177. (A, B, C, D) Adrenalectomy may be performed for many reasons, such as hypersecretion of adrenal hormones, neoplasms, or secondary treatment for neoplasms located elsewhere in the body. REF. 20, p. 194

178. (E) Cysts of the pancreas have been classified as follows: congenital, inflammatory, traumatic, neoplastic, or parasitic. REF. 20, p. 194

179. (C) The skin surface is the most common site of staphylococci. Studies have shown that up to 70% of persons carry this microorganism on their skin, which may lead to contamination of clothing and the shedding of microorganisms. REF. 20, p. 41

180. (E) Diplococcus pneumoniae is nonmotile, nonsporeforming, and produces no toxins of real significance. REF. 20, p. 42

181. (A) Gaseous gangrene is produced by spores of the Clostridium species present in contaminated wounds, especially those involving fracture or tissue necrosis. REF. 20, p. 43

182. (A) Escherichia coli is one of the most common causes of septicemia and inflammation of the urinary tract. However, most strains of E. coli are nonpathogenic in the normal healthy individual. REF. 20, p. 43

183. (C) Salmonella infections are acquired by ingestion of the microorganism, usually in contaminated food or water. REF. 20, p. 43

184. (B) Syphilis is caused by a spirochete, Treponema pallidum, that gains entry into the body through either the mucous membrane or skin during intercourse. REF. 35, p. 1448

185. (A,B,C) Numerous disease processes are linked with Staphylococcus aureus. The portals of entry are the skin, respiratory tract, and genitourinary tract. Pathogenic staphylococcus grows in sweat, urine, tissue, and skin. REF. 20, p. 41

186. (B) When infectious agents spread throughout the body tissues, the condition is termed a systemic infection. REF. 20, p. 40

187. (B) Resident microorganisms are those which habitually live in the epidermis, deep in the crevices and folds of the skin. REF. 20, p. 39

188. (C) N. gonorrhoeae gains entrance to the tissues after being deposited on and by burrowing through the mucous membranes. It then spreads via the lymphatic chain or blood vessels. REF. 20, p. 42

189. (A, B, C) Frequent washing of hands and proper handling and decontamination of all patient articles, tissue, and fluids can aid in preventing the spread of streptococcal infection. REF. 20, p. 42

190. (C) Evisceration is the extrusion of internal organs or viscera through a gaping wound. REF. 20, p. 127

191. (C) Inflammation is a defense reaction of the body to an injury or abnormal stimulation caused by a physical, chemical, or biological agent. REF. 20, p. 40

192. (D) The five cardinal symptoms of inflammation are redness, (rubor), heat due to hyperemia, swelling due to fluid exudate, pain due to irritation of nerve endings, and loss of function of affected part due to above. REF. 35, p. 179

193. (A, B) First intention healing occurs in wounds made aseptically with minimum tissue destruction and tissue reaction during the healing process. REF. 20, p. 125

194. (E) This type of wound is usually left open and allowed to heal from the inside out. It usually involves a wound that is infected or one where there is excessive loss of tissue and skin edges cannot be approximated. REF. 20, p. 125

195. (A, C) Healing by third intention implies that suturing is delayed for the purpose of walling off an area of gross infection. REF. 20, p. 125

196. (A) During the first 3-4 days of healing the incised tissue is held together by strands of fibrin and a thin layer of clotted blood. Plasma seeps to the surface to form a protective crust. REF. 20, p. 125

197. (B) After 3-4 days, connective tissue cells rapidly proliferate and give strength to the wound. As wound healing progresses, fibroblasts and capillaries greatly diminish in number. REF. 20, p. 125

198. (D) Immunity is provided when the external and internal defense mechanisms serve as the barrier excluding or destroying the invading agent. REF. 35, p. 170

199. (B) Sepsis is a generalized reaction to pathogenic microorganisms, their poisons, or both. REF. 20, p. 40

200. (A, B, C) The term contamination refers to the presense of pathogenic microorganisms on or in an animate or inanimate vector. REF. 20, p. 40

201. (C) Infection is the process by which living pathogenic microorganisms enter the body of the host under favorable conditions and produce toxins that may act injuriously on the tissues of the host. REF. 20, p. 39

202. (A) Natural immunity, a more or less permanent immunity to disease with which an individual is born, is the result of inherent factors. REF. 43, p. 710

203. (A) Passive immunity is acquired in utero from antibodies that pass from the mother to the fetus through the placenta or can be produced by injection of antibodies into the subject being protected. REF. 43, p. 710

204. (A, B, D) The basic principles of aseptic technique prevent contamination of open wounds. Isolate the operative site from the unsterile physical environment and create and maintain a sterile field in which to perform surgery in a safe manner. REF. 20, p. 46

205. (B) Bactericide is an agent that destroys bacteria but not necessarily their spores. REF. 43, p. 156

206. (A) Suppuration is the process of pus formation. REF. 43, p. 1393

207. (B) To provide protection from cross-contamination, all instruments should be terminally washed and sterilized after use and before being returned to trays or storage. REF. 20, p. 51

208. (A, D) A procedure is septic when there is known pathogenic bacteria or the presence of pus at the time of the procedure or known to surgeon prior to the procedure. REF. 20, p. 40

209. (A, C, D) Aseptic practices form the basis of sound surgical conscience.

210. (A, B, C) Each institution must determine its own procedures for OR apparel and standards according to accepted traffic patterns, finances available, and other factors. Within these constraints, each OR site maintains the highest possible standards. REF. 22, p. 416

211. (B) Semmelweis made a simple but important contribution to infection control by advocating that hands be washed between examinations of patients. REF. 20, p. 38

212. (C) In 1867 Lister was advocating carbolic soaks and sprays for hands, wounds, dressings, sutures, and the OR itself. REF. 20, p. 38

213. (E) All persons who enter restricted surgical areas should be required to wear clean OR apparel (IYFPA approved) consisting of head cover, shoe covers, masks, and one-piece or two-piece pantsuit or dress. REF. 20, p. 44

214. (B, C) An object or substance is considered sterile when it is completely free of all microorganisms and is incapable of producing any form of life. REF. 20, p. 46

215. (B) Cloth and gauze masks have a very low filtration efficiency and may become ineffective as a bacterial barrier within 30 min of wear. REF. 20, p. 46

216. (B, C) The sterility of bottle contents cannot be ensured if the cap is replaced on the bottle. After a sterile package is opened, the edges are considered unsterile. Sterile and unsterile boundaries are often intangible. REF. 20, p. 48

217. (A, B, C) When pouring solution into a sterile receptacle, the circulating nurse must maintain a safe margin of space to avoid contamination of sterile surfaces. REF. 20, p. 50

218. (B) The primary reason for the use of shoe covers is sanitation. When the same shoes are worn for successive operations, they provide a high bacterial count with the potential for cross-infection. REF. 20, p. 8

219. (C) A synthetic disposable mask should have an efficiency rate of at least 95%. In order for the mask to be effective, it must be worn correctly and handled properly. REF. 20, p. 46

220. (A, B, C, D) No jewelry should be worn in the OR, with the exception of pierced earring posts. REF. 20, p. 46

221. (A) An antiseptic is an agent capable of producing antisepsis. Chemically, antiseptics may be inorganic, such as mercury preparation, or organic, such as phenol. REF. 43, p. 99

222. (E) A disinfectant is a chemical which kills bacteria. The term is usually applied to a chemical or physical agent that kills vegetative forms of microorganisms. REF. 43, p. 416

223. (B) A bacteriostatic agent is an agent that inhibits or retards bacterial growth. REF. 43, p. 156

224. (A) A spore usually possesses a thick wall, enabling the cell to withstand unfavorable environmental conditions. REF. 43, p. 1351

225. (C) Sanitation is the application of measures to promote and establish conditions favorable to health. REF. 43, p. 1272

226. (A) Sterilization is the process of completely removing or destroying all microorganisms on a substance by exposure to chemical or physical agents. REF. 43, p. 1365

227. (D) The efficiency of a sterilization process depends on the kind of foreign material present, the number of instruments in the load, and are there more than one piece to each instrument and the material they are made of. REF. 20, p. 51

228. (A) Steam under pressure permits permeation of moist heat to porous substances by condensation and results in destruction of all microbial life. REF. 20, p. 52

229. (B) The high pressure instrument steam sterilizer is adjusted to operate at 270° F and 27 psi. The higher the steam pressure, the higher the temperature becomes. REF. 20, p. 57

230. (A) If the mixture of steam to air is changed the air acts as a barrier to steam penetration. 17-20 psi will be 250° F.

231. (D) Bacterial spores are the most resistant due to their thick protective wall surrounding the bacteria. REF: 43, p. 1351.

232. (E) Mechanical controls such as thermometers and automatic control assist in identifying and preventing malfunctions of the sterilizing equipment and operational errors made by personnel. REF. 20, p. 55

233. (A, D) In a gravity displacement sterilizer, instruments wrapped in 4 thickness of muslin should be exposed for 15 min at 270 F or 30 min at 250 F. REF. 20, p. 54

234. (D) In a gravity displacement sterilizer, instruments in an unwrapped perforated tray should be exposed for 3 min at 270 F. REF. 20, p. 54

235. (A) The efficiency of a washer sterilizer process depends on the kind of foreign material present and the number of open instruments being placed in the sterilizer. REF. 20, p. 54

236. (A) The "hivac" steam sterilizer speeds up the evacuation of air by drawing a partial vacuum in the chamber at the beginning of the cycle which removes the air. REF. 22, p. 213

237. (B) When gas sterilization is used, the agent is called ethylene oxide (EO), which is a highly toxic gas that can pollute the working environment. REF. 22, p. 215

238. (A, E) The hazards associated with EO have been greatly reduced by diluting the EO with inert gases such as carbon dioxide or freon. REF. 20, p. 58

239. (E) All items must be thoroughly cleaned and dried prior to EO sterilization so that no visible droplets remain. This is to allow proper formation of ethylene glycol for proper sterilization. REF. 20, p. 61

240. (E) EO is flammable and expensive but necessary for those items which are heat-, labile-, and moisture-sensitive. REF. 20, p. 58

241. (A, C, D) When EO-sterilized items are removed from the sterilizer, they should be transferred immediately to the aerator or aeration area. The length of aeration required is based on item composition. REF. 20, p. 261

242. (D) Radiation sterilization, or electron beam, is used widely in the medical device industry. The radiation passes through an entire product, killing organisms. No radioactive residue is left. REF. 22, pp. 216-217

243. (A, B, C) The most commonly used chemical disinfectants are 2% glutaraldehyde solution and phenolic combinations.

These solutions produce disinfection, but all chemicals are not safe for all devices. REF. 22, p. 217

244. (C) Mercurials are poor disinfectants and have no place in modern surgical disinfection. REF. 20, p. 63

245. (D) Lysol is a proprietary preparation of a mixture of cresols. Cresols are yellowish-brown liquids obtained from coal tar containing not more than 5% phenol. REF. 43, p. 845

246. (A, D) Phenol, when used carefully, is an effective bacteriostatic agent. REF. 43, p. 1088

247. (A, B, C) Chlorine preparations are used for disinfecting compounds (hypochlorites), such as Dakin's solution, or Javelle water, and are very effective in their germicidal power. REF. 43, p. 277

248. (B) Zephiran is a proprietary name for refined benzalkonium chloride. REF. 43, p. 1587

249. (E) The combination of polyvinylpyrolidone and iodine is the newest antiseptic agent used for skin disinfection. It possesses the potent germicidal effect of iodine without many of its irritating properties. REF. 20, p. 64

250. (A, B) An aqueous solution of formaldehyde is highly germicidal and sporicidal. Formaldehyde is also toxic to tissues and all materials treated with formaldehyde must be thoroughly rinsed before use. REF. 20, p. 64

251. (C) Cidex is a 2% glutaraldehyde solution.

252. (C) Many disinfectants are corrosive to metals and rubber. They are irritating to tissue. Therefore, all items must be rinsed thoroughly to prevent damage to items or skin. REF. 20, pp. 63-64

253. (A, B) Packing of surgical supplies and their arrangement in loads in the sterilizer are important factors that govern the effectiveness of steam sterilization. REF. 20, pp. 53-55

254. (C) Every package intended for sterile use should be labelled with a control number that identifies the date of

sterilization, sterilizer used, cycle or load number, and the date of expiration. REF. 20, p. 54

255. (A,B) The size and density of woven textile packs must be restricted to ensure uniform steam penetration. Packs should be wrapped sequentially in two double-thickness wrappers or the equivalent in other types of wrappers. The familiar envelope wrap should be used for presentation. REF. 20, p. 53

256. (A,C,D) Muslin wraps must be a 140 thread count, laundered between sterilization exposures, and checked for holes before they are used. REF. 20, p. 53

257. (A,B,C) Textile materials are treated with a chemical that renders them highly resistant to liquid penetration. REF. 43, p. 211

258. (A,C,D) Shelf-life is the result of the interrelationship of the following conditions: packaging, sterilization, handling, and storage. Guidelines followed in most institutions are: double-wrapped muslin, 21-30 days; heat-sealed or enclosed with dust covers, 6 months-1 year. REF. 20, p. 55

259. (A, B, C) All muslin wrappers must be inspected for tears and holes, items within pack must be assembled to allow for proper steam penetration, and a wrapped cycle should be used to allow for adequate sterilization (250° F 30 min).

260. (A, B) Orthopedic instruments, equipment, and appliances require special care, storage, and handling. Appropriate sterilization cases should be used. Sterilization procedures are according to manufacturer's instructions. REF. 20, p. 461

261. (E) Dry heat is the method of choice for powders and oils that cannot be sterilized by steam or retain ethylene oxide or its byproducts. REF. 22, p. 216

262. (C) Instruments wrapped in four thicknesses of muslin should be exposed for 15 min at 270° F or 30 min at 250° F. REF. 20, p. 54

263. (C) Items to be ethylene oxide sterilized must be thoroughly cleaned and towel or air dried so no visible droplets remain. REF. 20, p. 61

III. Care of the Patient

264. (C) Preparation of the patient, both physically and psychologically, to withstand the effects of anesthesia and surgery is accomplished by parts one and two of the nursing process: assessment and planning. REF. 20, p. 4

265. (D) Patients express their anxiety by many behavioral manifestations, including open hostility, aggression, indifference, and excessive talking.

266. (B,D,E) Preoperative medications should produce a desirable physical state of decreased tension and anxiety, and decreased salivations and bronchial secretions. Reactions of profuse perspiration, dizziness, and headache would be considered adverse in nature.

267. (B,D,E) When transporting patients to the OR, the transporter first reports to the nurse or person in charge at the desk, picks up the chart, and proceeds to the patient's room. He should introduce himself to the patient and check the patient's identification band. The stretcher should be locked in place and adequate personnel (at least two persons) available to help the patient move onto the stretcher.

268. (E)

269. (D) Skin preparation in the OR has the disadvantages that the patient's anesthesia time is prolonged, optimum use of the OR is infringed on, and loose hair remaining on the surrounding lines may get into the wound. REF. 20, p. 70

270. (A,C) In shaving the operative site, great care should be taken to avoid cutting or nicking the skin because cutaneous bacteria will proliferate in these areas. Nicks or cuts should be reported as incidents and the surgeon notified by the OR charge nurse. REF. 20, pp. 66, 70

271. (A) Based on the schedule and the operating surgeon's preference, the basic patient position is anticipated. REF. 20, p. 91

272. (A) The position at the head should place the cervical, thoracic, and lumbar vertebrae in a straight horizontal line. The arms should rest easily at the sides with the palms against the padded body or with the hands pronated (palms down and fingers extended) on the mattress surface. REF. 20, pp. 93, 94

273. (C,D,E) Trendelenburg is a variant of the basic supine position with the body tilted head down. The leg may be lowered parallel to the floor to maintain the position. This position is used either to provide better visualization of the pelvic organs or to improve circulation to the cerebral cortex and basal ganglia when blood pressure is suddenly lowered. REF. 20, pp. 95, 439

274. (A,C) Reverse Trendelenburg is frequently used to facilitate gravitational pull on the viscera away from the diaphragm and toward the feet. The patient's body must be supported by the padded footboard, by nonconstrictive body restraints, and by a lift sheet that supports the arms from elbows to fingers. REF. 20, p. 96

275. (A,B,C) The backrest is elevated, the knees are flexed, and the footboard is set in place. The sitting position requires special attention to positioning of the arms. This position is used primarily in neurosurgical procedures. REF. 20, pp. 96, 443

276. (E) By placing the patient's anterior iliac spine on a line with the leg holder and the buttocks level and on a line with the edge of the table break, a good position can be achieved with a minimum of effort. The stirrups must be level. To place a patient in the lithotomy position, the patient's legs are raised simultaneously. The arms may be folded loosely across the abdomen so as not to impede chest movement and adequate respiration. REF. 20, pp. 96-97

277. (E) In the lateral position, the patient is lying on the unaffected side, and the surgical approach may be to the uppermost chest, the kidney, or the upper ureter. The hazards of neuromuscular damage can largely be prevented

through careful manipulation and adequate protective padding. REF. 20, pp. 98, 100

278. (B,D) After the anesthetized patient is turned from the dorsal position to the lateral position, he is moved so that the lower iliac crest is just below the kidney elevator of the table. The table is then flexed to lower his head and legs. REF. 20, p. 99

279. (E) Modifications of the position allow approach to the cervical spine, back, rectal area, and lower extremities. The jackknife or Kraske's position is a modification of the prone position. The head is positioned, keeping the neck in alignment with the spinal column. The eyes are carefully protected from pillows and drapes. The respiratory system is most vulnerable because the normal anterolateral respiratory movement is restricted and the normal diaphragmatic movement is inhibited by the compressed abdominal wall. A pillow placed under the ankles prevents pressure on the toes and plantar phexiva of the feet. Neuromuscularly, the radial nerve may be compressed against the humerus if the forearm is allowed to hang over the side of the table. REF. 20, p. 97

280. (B,C,E) An effective anesthetic will produce a state of sleep, provide analgesia, obtain adverse reflexes, and relax muscles. REF. 20, p. 157

281. (D) Inhalational agents are desirable because of their ease of uptake and elimination through the respiratory system. Many agents may be given intravenously to cause a safe, reversible state of anesthesia. Topical anesthesia is the direct application of anesthetic drugs to skin or mucous surfaces. REF. 22, pp. 157-160

282. (A) Four stages of anesthesia are classically described with ether anesthesia, but they are virtually the same for all anesthetic agents. Stage 1 begins with the patient awake and continues to loss of consciousness. Stage 2 is from loss of consciousness during which the patient begins automatic breathing, following which excitement occurs with irregular breathing and limb movement. Stage 3 is heralded by regular respirations and is the the stage of surgical anesthesia. Stage 4 is apnea leading to death. REF. 22, pp. 160-161

283. (A,B,E) Local anesthetic agents primarily exert their action by inhibition of the excitatory process in nerve endings or nerve fibers. A drug commonly used for infiltration and local injection anesthesia is 0. 5-2% lidocaine (Xylocaine) with or without epinephrine. The patient does not lose consciousness and is aware of the surroundings. REF. 22, pp. 33, 134

284. (B,D) The most frequently used anesthetic agents are lidocaine and chloroprasaise. The injected local anesthetic bathes the nerve roots as they leave the cord through the intervertebral foramina, blocking conduction of impulses through them. REF. 20, p. 138

285. (A) Spinal anesthesia is obtained by introducing local anesthetics into the subarachnoid space. REF. 22, p. 160

286. (E) Lists for CPR. REF. 20, pp. 36-37.

287. (A, B, C) For the total protection of the surgical patient, it is imperative that the surgical team know intimately the location of all emergency equipment available. REFS. 20, pp. 36-37; 22, pp. 354-356

288. (B,D,E) Hazards can be controlled by installing explosion-proof switches and motors, use of conductive flooring, and proper clothing by personnel. REFS. 20, pp. 30-31; 22, pp. 163-167

289. (B,C) Operating rooms should have at least 25 room air exchanges per hour, five changes of which should be fresh air. Positive pressure and high-efficiency particulator air filters are routinely being used. REF. 20, p. 26

IV. Operating Room Techniques

290. (A,B) As a patient advocate, the OR personnel have as one of their most important functions establishing and maintaining asepsis during the intraoperative phase of surgery. It is imperative that a "surgical conscience" be developed that allows no compromises in the principles of asepsis and sterile technique. REF. 22, p. 409

291. (E) All items used within a sterile field should be sterile. Any items of questionable sterility should be

considered unsterile. The entire team is alert to breaks in technique and quick to make corrections. REF. 22, pp. 411, 430

292. (A,B,E) Drapes must be resistant to moisture strike-through, safe, and easily drapable. The patient and operating table are covered with sterile drapes in a manner that exposes the prepared site of incision and isolates the area of the surgical wound. The variety of drapes should be kept to a minimum, simple, and economical in terms of time, body motions, and materials. REFS. 20, pp. 84-85; 22, p. 428

293. (E) Several types of impermeable polyvinyl sheeting are available; they facilitate draping of irregular body surfaces, form a complete seal over the skin at the site of incision, and prevent skin excretions and bacteria from coming in contact with the wound. Skin color and anatomical landmarks are readily visible. REF. 20, p. 85

294. (D) Transient bacteria are usually limited to exposed areas of skin. REF. 22

295. (D,E) All nails and subungual spaces are cleansed with a disposable nail cleaner. REF. 20, p. 73

296. (A) The timed scrub will usually take at least 5 min to complete. REF. 22, p. 417

297. (A,C,E) The gown should be grasped firmly at the neckline and allowed to unfold completely, with the inside of the gown toward the wearer. The person inserts both arms simultaneously, with the circulator assisting by pulling the gown up over the shoulders of the scrub person, touching only the inner aspect of the gown. REFS. 20, p. 76; 22, p. 420

298. (A,C,D) An unscrubbed person should untie the gown in the back. The scrub person then grasps the gown's shoulders on the outside, pulls item down over the arms, and then completely down over the gloved hands. REF. 22, p. 425

299. (A,C,D) The closed method of gloving has the advantage of preventing the bare hands from coming in contact with the outside of the sterile glove. The hands are pushed

through the cuff openings as the gloves are pulled in place. REF. 20, p. 79

300. (A,C) The glove is grasped under the inverted cuff. The cuff is stretched to open the glove. REF. 20, p. 82

301. (B) Chemically treated cotton cloth and tightly woven 100% cotton cloth with an appropriate thread count of 288/sq in. provide a barrier to liquids and are abrasion resistant. REF. 20, p. 84

302. (E) The disposable drapes currently on the market are soft, lint free, lightweight, compact, flame and moisture resistant, nonirritating, and static free. REF. 20, p. 84

303. (E) A whole or plain sheet is used to cover instrument tables, operating tables, and body regions. Slit sheets are used for draping patients, leaving the operative site exposed. A laparotomy sheet is large enough to cover the patient, operating table and extend over the anesthesia screen. The perineal sheet is used for operations on the perineum and genitalia. REF. 20, p. 85

304. (E) Drapes should not be slipped, fanned, or shaken. If a towel clip has been secured through a drape, it cannot be moved as it must be considered contaminated. If the sterility of a drape is questionable, it must be considered contaminated. REF. 20, pp. 88, 89

305. (E) Between surgical procedures, personnel must remove their gowns and gloves and place them in the proper receptacles. All linen should be discarded in linen hamper bags. Used disposable items should be discarded in plastic bags. Wet linen should be placed in the center of the bundle to prevent soaking through to the outside of the bag. REF. 20, p. 89

306. (E) Assessment is the collection of relevant data about the patient by preoperative interview with the patient and the patient's family and by review of the patient's chart for past medical/surgical history. Assessment is knowing and understanding the patient as a person and as a candidate for a surgical procedure. REF. 20, p. 4

307. (A,C,D) The operative consent form, history, and physical and laboratory examination results should be complete.

These usually include recent determinations of blood and urine and chest x-ray examination. REF. 20, p. 30

308. (C) The OR nurse should review the patient's identification band. REF. 20, p. 30

309. (B, C) Opiates such as morphine and Demerol reduce the amount of general anesthesia required. Anticholinergics relax smooth muscle, inhibit secretions of duct glands, and prevent laryngospasm. REF. 22, p. 145

310. (A) Temperature should be controlled at between 20 and 24° C (68 and 75° F). REF. 20, p. 25

311. (C) Humidity should be controlled at a minimum of 50% to aid in the control of bacterial growth and the suppression of static electricity. REF. 20, p. 25

312. (E) It is important to check the following: inadequate patient contact with the plate, poor placement of the plate, inadequate connection of the cable to the plate, and inadequate connection of the unit. REF. 20, p. 32

313. (A, B, D) Kinks and curls should be removed from electrical cords before plugging into wall outlets. Wire and connections should be handled in accordance with their delicacy to prevent cord breakage. Personnel must receive instruction in the safe usage of all equipment. All electrical equipment must be checked before a surgical procedure begins. REF. 20, p. 31

314. (E) Effective hospital and OR infection control programs must be carried out by all persons who help care for patients. These programs include strict aseptic technique and sterility of surgical equipment. All members of the surgical team have a duty to protect the patient from any deleterious effects of the surgical position. Personnel must receive instruction in the safe usage of all equipment. REF. 20, pp. 38, 91, 31

315. (E) Modern operating tables are specifically designed to meet the peculiar and highly specialized requirements of surgical therapy. Many accessory parts are included. REF. 22, pp. 346-348

316. (B, D, E) Counting is part of the professional nurse's responsibility for patient safety. Estimation of blood loss

is a vital procedure in the surgical management of all patients. REFS. 20, p. 34; 22, p. 457

317. (A,C,D) After surgery, a dressing may be applied to the wound; some drains are taped or sutured into place and others are attached to or function by way of continuous or intermittent vacuum and suction. At a minimum, there should be four individuals transferring the patient from operating table to stretcher or bed.

318. (A,C) Every surgical wound is considered to be potentially contaminated. A broad-spectrum detergent/germicide should be used in the efficient and thorough cleaning of the OR. REF. 20, pp. 89-90

319. (A,D) The floor should be cleaned with a detergent/germicide using the wet vacuum method. REF. 20, p. 90

320. (A,C,D) Mammal suture can be absorbable, such as chromic or plain catgut. REF. 22, p. 361

321. (B,C) Fine cotton sutures, when buried in tissue, produce minimum tissue reaction; nylon is nonirritating to tissues. Both can be used for internal suturing.

322. (A,C,D) The uses of surgical stainless steel are widespread; it has strength, inertness, and low tissue reaction. It ranges in sizes from 7 to 6-0 or B&S gauge 18 to 40. REF. 20, p. 105

323. (B) The most popular needle type is the swaged or atraumatic needle. REF. 20, p. 111

324. (A,B,D) A retention or stay suture is placed at a distance from the primary suture line and is usually of a heavy, nonabsorbable material. REF. 20, p. 110

325. (B,C) Examples of polypropylene suture material are proline and surgilene. REF. 20, p. 105

326. (A,B,C) Examples of synthetic polyamide material are Dermalon, Surgilon, and Nurolon. REF. 20, p. 104

327. (C) Suture ligature is a strand of suture material threaded or swaged on a needle. REF. 20, p. 106

328. (C) A ligature is a strand used to encircle or close off the lumen of a vessel. REF. 20, p. 106

329. (C) The LDS is used to ligate and divide omental vessels. REF. 20, p. 107

330. (A,B,D) Suture needles vary in shape, size, point design, and wire diameter; they are strong enough to pass through tissue without causing trauma. REF. 20, p. 111

331. (B,C) Surgical needles fall into three general categories, two of which have threaded eyes. The shaft of the needle is the needle body. REF. 20, p. 111

332. (E) Types and sizes of sponges should be kept at a minimum, counted carefully, and should be nontraumatic and x-ray detectable. REF. 20, p. 34

333. (A,B,D) The circulating nurse counts the sponges before beginning the operation, before the closure begins, and after skin closure is started. Additional counts should be taken according to individual hospital policy and circumstances. REF. 20, p. 34

334. (B,C,D) Drains are usually placed to provide an exit through which air and fluids, such as serum and blood, can be evacuated. In some instances, drainage is directly through a tube, such as in the chest cavity to remove air. Some drains drain independently. REF. 20, p. 130

335. (A,C) The Malecot four-winged catheter is often used as a nephrostomy tube to provide temporary or permanent diversion of urine. A Foley catheter may also be used for this purpose. REF. 20, p. 246

336. (B) A type of sump drain is usually used in areas with a large amount of drainage and is attached to or functions by way of systems of continuous or intermittent vacuum or suction.

337. (B) A gastrostomy tube is a temporary or permanent channel or tube placed in the gastric lumen and brought out of the abdomen through a separate stab wound. REF. 20, p. 217

338. (B,C) Pleurovac system is a compact, disposable unit for drainage of the chest after surgery. Another closed, portable, self-contained drainage system is the Hemovac. REF. 20, pp. 356, 129

339. (E) No dressing on the operative site allows for optimal observation of the incisional area, prevents possible adhesive tape reactions, increases maneuverability of the patient, and minimizes adverse responses to the operation by the patient. REF. 20, p. 128

340. (B) If frequent dressings are anticipated, the dressing may be secured with Montgomery straps. REF. 20, p. 128

341. (D) The scrub nurse pulls the suture about 4 in. through the eye of the needle. REF. 20, p. 112

342. (B) If a drainage tube is inserted in the wound, a tube may be anchored to the skin with a nonabsorbable suture. REF. 20, p. 110

343. (A,C) Sharps are instruments used for cutting, such as scissors and scalpels. Clamping instruments are for hemostasis. Grasping instruments are used for tissue retraction or suturing, and retractors determine the exposure of the operative field. REF. 20, pp. 116-119

344. (B) Metzenbaum scissors are used for dissection of delicate tissues. REF. 20, p. 116

345. (C) Bandage scissors would be used for dissection of heavy tissue seen in cesarean sections. REF. 20, p. 116

346. (C) Mixter clamps are often referred to as right angle clamps. REF. 20, p. 185 (Figure 13-4, #3)

347. (C) Lahey forceps are commonly used for heavy tissue and specimen grasping. REF. 20, p. 185 (Figure 13-4 #4)

348. (B,D) Babcock clamps have curved, fenestrated blades with no teeth and grip or enclose delicate structures. REF. 20, pp. 117, 119

349. (A,C) Payr pylorus clamps are used for intestinal and gastric surgery. REF. 20, p. 211

350. (A,C,D) Retractors can be self-retaining: an example is the Witlaner, which has two blades held apart by a racket. It comes in three sizes and is a superficial tissue retractor. REF. 20, pp. 119, 120 (Figure 7-26)

351. (B) An Aunard weighted speculum would be used on vaginal or cervical procedures. REF. 20, p. 312 (Figure 16-11)

352. (C,E) A Graves speculum is used on procedures involving the vagina and cervix. REF. 20, p. 312 (Figure 16-11)

353. (B) A Satinsky clamp is found in the instrument set-up for cardiovascular surgery. REF. 20, p. 389 (Figure 18-13)

354. (D) Hank dilators are used in surgery on the uterine cervix. REF. 20, p. 313 (Figure 16-12)

355. (B) Vulsellum tenaculi are found in the set-up for surgery of the uterus. REF. 20, p. 312 (Figure 16-10)

356. (C,D) Bull dog clamps, designed to occlude blood flow, may be straight, curved, or adjustable spring-type. REF. 20, p. 389

357. (C,E) The Alexander costal periosteotome, included in instrumentation for rib resection or thoracic set-up, is used to free the intercostal muscles from the rib. REF. 20, pp. 359, 361

358. (E) The Gaylor biopsy forcep is an accessory item of the basic vaginal set-up. REF. 20, pp. 311, 313

359. (C) The Yankauer suction tip is an accessory item for laparotomy instrumentation and is used for many procedures requiring suction. REF. 20, pp. 147, 539, 638

360. (D) The Castroviejo caliper is included in the instrumentation for eye examination and for eye muscle operations. REF. 20, pp. 674, 692

361. (B) Gouges are included in the basic set of bone instruments. REF. 20, p. 462

362. (B) Doyen rib raspatories, used to free the intercostal muscles from the rib, are included in instrumentation for rib resection or thoracotomy. REF. 20, pp. 359, 361

363. (D) The Gigli saw, or air-powered craniotome, is used to cut between burr holes in the skull. REF. 2, p. 434

364. (C) Bethune rib shears are included in instrumentation for thoracotomy. REF. 20, p. 360

365. (A) The Ferris-Smith knife dermatome is used to obtain grafts in a "freehand" manner. REF. 20, p. 533

366. (B) Kerrison rongeurs are included in basic instrumentation for supratentorial craniotomy and laminectomy. REF. 20, pp. 736, 765

367. (A) Mayo common duct scoops, Mayo cystic duct scoops, and Moore gall stone scoops are included in instrumentation for biliary surgery. REF. 20, p. 185

368. (C) A Hill retractor, or rectal speculum, would be used in a hemorrhoidectomy procedure. REF. 16, pp. 241, 242

369. (B) The Jackson forceps is designed for foreign body removal from the larynx, trachea, bronchi, esophagus, or mediastinum. REF. 20, p. 362

370. (E) Important instrument checks include: jaw and teeth should be in alignment; ratchets should hold firmly, yet release easily; tips of jaws and teeth should meet perfectly; and scissors should be sharp. REF. 20, p. 124

371. (C) Ultrasonic waves form small bubbles that expand until they are unstable and then collapse quickly, creating a negative pressure action on all surfaces of instruments in the bath. REF. 20, p. 52

372. (A,B) Long, narrow brushes and long pipe cleaners should be available for cleaning the lumen, suction, and light channels of endoscopes. REF. 20, p. 634

373. (B) All instruments, supplies, and equipment used in surgery must be either terminally sterilized, decontaminated, or contained for disposal before they are

handled by personnel to protect against contamination by known or unknown organisms. REF. 2, p. 153

374. (A,C) Ligation clips can be placed around vessels, nerves, or ducts via a special applicator. The clips are available in various sizes in cartridge form. REF. 16, p. 129

375. (E) Resection, transection, and anastomoses can all be accomplished with various stapling instruments which employ fine stainless staples formed into a "B" shape. REF. 16, p. 129

376. (B,C,E) OR nurses and technologists are responsible for proper cleaning, maintenance, and assembly of stapling instruments. Preparation for use includes knowing the technique for loading the cartridge and anvil. Proper placement of safety locks prevents premature firing of the instrument. REF. 16, pp. 129-134

377. (E) Eye surgical instrumentation includes the Jameson muscle hook, Barraquer needle holder, Jaeger retractor, and McPherson speculum. REF. 16, pp. 178, 179

378. (C) Cushing elevators used in neurosurgery may be sharp, small, and blunt or wide with a square edge. REF. 16, p. 173

379. (A,B,C) The Aufrich retractor, Hartmann dressing forceps, and Joseph button knife are used for nasal surgery. REF. 16, pp. 184-187

380. (A,C,D) Instruments to repair a torn meniscus or torn ligament of the knee would include the Stille-Luer rongeur, osteotomes, and short curettes. REF. 16, pp. 330, 333

381. (E) Skin preparation, treatment of known infections, segregating the patient's face from the open wound, and prevention of contamination when the bowel is open are all efforts to reduce the patient source of contamination. REF. 23, pp. 36, 37

382. (B,C,E) The scrub team source of contamination can be reduced by proper scrubbing, gowning, and gloving; covering all exposed hair; and not touching the patient's skin with sterile gloved hands. REF. 23, pp. 36, 37

383. (B,C,E) Standards of Practice considers all surgical wounds potentially contaminated and recommends that all items that come in contact with the patient and the sterile field should be discarded or terminally cleaned. Also, gloves or instruments should be used when collecting and counting sponges. In addition to cleaning between cases, terminal cleaning at the end of a day's schedule would include the wet vacuum method of floor care. REF. 1, pp. 14-16

V. Surgery

384. (C) The paramedian rectus incision can be used in any intra-abdominal surgery when on the appropriate side. REF. 20, p. 148

385. (A,D) The vertical midline incision is an excellent primary incision and is generally preferred because it offers good exposure to any part of the abdominal cavity. REF. 20, p. 148

386. (C) The Pfannenstiel incision is a curved transverse incision across the lower abdomen used frequently for gynecological surgery. REF. 20, p. 149

387. (B,C,D) The McBurney muscle-splitting incision is an oblique incision that begins well below the umbilicus, goes through the McBurney's point, and extends upward toward the right flank. It is used for removal of the appendix. REF. 20, pp. 148, 149

388. (E) The subcostal incision, made on the right, is sometimes preferred for operations on the gallbladder, common duct, or pancreas. If made on the left, it may be used for splenectomy. REF. 20, p. 149

389. (C) The thoracoabdominal incision begins at a midpoint between the xiphoid process and the umbilicus, extends across to the seventh or eighth interspace and to the midscapular line. The abdominal part may be made first for exploration, then if necessary extended across the costal margin into the chest. REF. 20, p. 150

390. (B,C) Surgical incisions should provide maximum exposure, be easily extended and closed, heal primarily, provide maximum postoperative wound strength, and

minimum postoperative wound discomfort. REF. 23, p. 174

391. (E) The right upper paramedian incision would be used for biliary tract surgery. REF. 23, p. 175

392. (A, D, E) The lower abdominal midline incision provides excellent exposure of the pelvic organs, is easily extended, and is quickly executed and closed. However, it lacks the strength of a transverse or lower paramedian incision. REF. 23, p. 175

393. (A, B, E) Fine sutures would be used for subcutaneous abdominal layers. Noncutting needles would be used for peritoneal closure. REF. 20, p. 147

394. (A, B, E) Included in the set-up for basic laparotomy opening are the following: accessory items such as Yankauer suction; cutting instruments such as #3, 4, and 7 knife handles; and exposing instruments, such as various retractors, including Kelly and Richardson. REF. 20, p. 143

395. (A, B) A congenital or acquired opening or fascial defect in the abdominal wall may allow displacement of intra-abdominal tissue or viscus. Thus, a hernia or sac lined by peritoneum may be pushed through the defect in the layers of abdominal wall. REF. 20, p. 152

396. (A) If the contents of the hernia sac can be returned to the normal intra-abdominal position, it is reducible; if they are trapped in the extra-abdominal sac, the hernia is incarcerated. REF. 20, p. 152

397. (A, B) Most hernias occur in the inguinal or femoral region. REF. 2, p. 330

398. (A, B) Most hernias involving bowel that reach the stage of vascular compromise do cause the signs and symptoms of intestinal obstruction and require immediate attention. REF. 38, p. 1337

399. (C) A simple mastectomy is removal of the entire involved breast without lymph node dissection. It is performed to remove extensive benign disease, if malignancy is believed to be confined only to the breast tissue,

or as a palliative measure in advanced malignancy. REF. 20, pp. 168-172

400. (C) Excision of a portion of a breast mass for pathological examination and estrogen-progesterone receptor assay is an incisional biopsy. Excisional biopsy is excision of the entire mass for examination. REF. 20, pp. 168-172

401. (E) X-ray mammography is a screening device for early breast cancer detection. Thermography and ultrasound should be used as an adjunct to physical exam and mammography. REF. 20, p. 167

402. (E) If malignant cells are encountered in an incisional breast biopsy and further surgery is to be performed, a change of instruments, drapes, gowns, and gloves may be required. REF. 20, p. 168

403. (A,B,C) Vein ligation and stripping requires skin incision in the groin and ankles. Major veins can be removed with internal strippers and accessory veins by direct incision. Following this procedure, a compression dressing is applied to the full length of the leg. REF. 20, p. 343

404. (C,D) Rectal surgery is performed in the prone, Buie, or Kraske position under general or spinal anesthesia. Identification of a fistulous tract may be aided by the use of dye or a probe and grooved director. Electrosurgery or cryosurgery may be used in rectal procedures such as hemorrhoidectomy or rectal tumors. REF. 2, pp. 329, 330

405. (C,D) Direct hernias occur within Hesselbach's triangle. Indirect hernias occur lateral to deep epigastric vessels. Both represent tears in the transversalis fascia. REF. 20, p. 153

406. (C) Varicosities are abnormally dilated veins. The vein most commonly affected in the lower extremities is the long saphenous vein. REF. 8, p. 477

407. (A,B) Treatment of varicosities may include high ligation and division of the saphenous trunk with or without subsequent stripping and excision. REF. 20, p. 443

408. (A,C,D) A hemorrhoidectomy is defined as surgical excision and ligation of varicosities of the anus and rectum that do not respond to conservative treatment. REF. 2, p. 329

409. (A,C) An appendectomy is the removal and severance of the appendix from its attachment to the cecum, through a right lower quadrant muscle-splitting or McBurney incision. Following dissection of the mesoappendix from the appendiceal wall, a purse string suture is placed in the cecal wall at the base of the appendix. If the appendix has ruptured, the peritoneum is drained and a Penrose or suction drain left in place. The wound may be packed open to allow healing by secondary intent. REF. 20, p. 225

410. (A,C,D) Cholecystectomy, removal of the gallbladder, is performed through a right subcostal, right paramedian, or midline incision. A cholecystectomy requires that the cystic duct and artery are divided, ligated, and transfixed with suture. It also requires that the common bile duct be identified and not injured. REF. 20, pp. 184-187

411. (E) <u>Cholecystojejunostomy</u> is the establishment of continuity by an anastomosis between the gallbladder and jejunum to relieve an obstruction in the distal end of the common duct. <u>Choledochojejunostomy</u> is an anastomosis between the common duct and the jejunum. <u>Cholecystoduodenostomy</u> is the establishment of continuity by an anastomosis between the gallbladder and duodenum. <u>Choledochoduodenostomy</u> is an anastomosis between the common duct and the duodenum. REF. 20, pp. 184-187

412. (D) The suture the surgeon might use to sew the gallbladder bed would be 3-0 chromic with a small taper needle. Following removal of the gallbladder, all bleeding is controlled and reperitonealization of the gallbladder bed, if indicated, is accomplished with interrupted or continuous fine chromic intestinal sutures. REF. 20, p. 187

413. (E) If choledocholithiasis or an obstruction of the common bile duct is suspected, a cholangiogram may be scheduled. An x-ray table with cassette, radiopaque dye, cholangiogram catheters, Bakes dilators, probes, scoops, Mixters, and assorted sizes of T tubes should be considered for this procedure. REF. 20, pp. 184-189

414. (A, C) Repair of strictures of the common and hepatic ducts for relief of biliary obstruction may be accomplished by resection of the stricture and an end-to-end anastomosis over a T-tube splint or by means of anastomosis between the duct and the intestinal tract. REF. 20, p. 192

415. (E) A Whipple procedure or pancreaticoduodenectomy includes removal of the head of the pancreas, the entire duodenum, a portion of the jejunum, the distal third of the stomach, and the lower half of the common bile duct with reestablishment of continuity of the biliary, pancreatic, and GI systems. REF. 20, p. 194

416. (E) Consideration for hepatic resection should include facilities for hypothermia, electrocoagulation, measuring portal pressure, thoracotomy drainage, accurate replacement of blood loss, and special needles for suturing liver tissue. REF. 20, pp. 196, 197

417. (B) If the GI tract is entered, bowel technique must be used. This means that any instrument coming in contact with the GI mucosa is not used after the lumen of the GI tract has been restored. These instruments are discarded in a separate basin and do not come in contact with other instruments. REF. 20, pp. 210, 211

418. (E) Strictures in the lower esophagus may develop after trauma, infection, or corrosion or because of the presence of tumors. REF. 20, p. 212

419. (C) Pyloroplasty forms a larger passageway between the prepyloric region of the stomach and the first or second portion of the duodenum, with excision of peptic ulcer, if present. REF. 20, p. 216

420. (E) The Hickman catheter or infusaid pump may be implanted to assist in administration of chemotherapy, pain-controlling agents, hyperalimentation, or antibiotics. REF. 7, pp. 1335-1368

421. (D, E) The single-tooth tenaculum and Heaney forceps are instruments for gynecological surgery. REF. 20, pp. 312, 314

422. (B,C,D) Instruments and materials used to enter bile ducts should be considered contaminated. X-rays are often used to locate or confirm removal of gallstones. Drains are commonly used after cholecystectomy or choledochotomy. Aspirating needle and syringe can be helpful to the surgeon in identifying bile ducts and arteries. REF. 20, pp. 184, 188, 189

423. (C,D) Choledochoscopy, direct visualization of the common bile duct by means of the choledochoscope, is performed via the operative procedure for choledochotomy. Saline is used to distend and flush the duct for visualization and irrigation. REF. 20, pp. 190, 191

424. (E) Splenectomy is most often performed for hypersplenism, causing a reduction in circulating red cells, white cells, or platelets. Other reasons for operative intervention include rupture, accessory spleens, or tumors. REF. 2, p. 324

425. (D) Mayo and Allen clamps are used in intestinal anastomosis. REF. 16, pp. 22, 221

426. (C) Current preferred treatment for chronic duodenal ulcer is the parietal or proximal cell vagotomy. REF. 3, pp. 4, 5

427. (A,B,C) Partial gastrectomy with gastroduodenostomy would require Allis or Babcock clamps to grasp the surface of the stomach and Kocher and Allen clamps for resection and anastomosis of the duodenum. REF. 16, p. 210

428. (C) Morbid obesity may be treated surgically by the gastric bypass, gastroplasty, or gastric-partitioning operations. REF. 39, pp. 1137, 1138

429. (A,B,C) The Koch pouch may be created instead of the conventional ileostomy following a proctocolectomy. A surgically constructed reservoir allows patients to control expulsion of feces and gas by emptying the pouch regularly through a stoma in the right lower quadrant. REF. 25, pp. 191-201

430. (C) An ileostomy may be done when an extensive lesion is present to provide complete rest of the colon by means

of diversion or when the entire large bowel is resected. REF. 20, p. 228

431. (B) A colostomy is performed to treat obstruction in the sigmoid colon. To decompress the bowel or to give the bowel a rest may necessitate a temporary colostomy. REF. 20, p. 228

432. (E) The abdominal perineal resection requires mobilization and division of diseased bowel through a midline incision. A colostomy is created by using the proximal end of the sigmoid. The distal end is removed through the perineum. This operation is performed for malignant and inflammatory lesions of the lower sigmoid colon, rectum, and anus. REF. 20, pp. 232, 233

433. (B,D) The submucous resection (SMR) is performed to improve the nasal airway by resecting a segment of septal cartilage. REF. 20, pp. 566, 567

434. (E) Some of the instruments included in the set-up for a submucous resection are cartilage knives, bayonet forceps, Freer elevator, Frazier suction tip, osteotomes, mallet, nasal saws, and double-action nasal rongeur. REF. 20, pp. 567, 568

435. (A,C,D) The intranasal antrostomy or antral window is an opening into the maxillary sinus through the nose with removal of accessory polyps and degenerated mucosa. The Caldwell-Luc or radical antrostomy approaches the maxillary sinus via an incision into the canine fossa of the upper jaw and exposure of the antrum, for removal of bony diseased portions of the antral wall and contents of the sinus or establishment of drainage and aeration. Ethmoidectomy is removal of the diseased portion of the middle turbinate, removal of ethmoidal cells, and removal of diseased tissue in the nasal fossa through a nasal or external approach. Removal of nasal polyps is often done in conjunction with these operations. REF. 20, pp. 624-628

436. (E) Instruments required to perform a tonsillectomy and adenoidectomy include the Jennings or McIvor mouth gag, adenoid curettes, Schnitz or tonsil hemostat, and Yankauer suction. REF. 20, p. 637

437. (E) Instruments added to the basic dissecting set for thyroid surgery include Lahey vulsellum forceps, Green retractors, Farr or spring retractors, self-retaining thyroid retractor, and straight and curved fine hemostats. REF. 20, p. 175

438. (B, C, D) Care must be taken throughout the thyroidectomy procedure to carefully identify and preserve the parathyroid glands, recurrent laryngeal nerve, and the jugular vein. REF. 20, pp. 177, 178

439. (E) The operative procedure for parotidectomy includes identification of the following important structures: the auricular nerve, the superficial temporal artery and vein, the external jugular vein, and the temporal, zygomatic, mandibular, and cervical branches of the facial nerve. REF. 20, p. 644

440. (E) Instruments and supplies necessary for laryngectomy and radical neck dissection include bone instruments (for division of the hyoid bone), suction and cautery equipment, many mosquito clamps, and laryngectomy tubes. REF. 20, pp. 648-650

441. (A, B, C) Equipment and instruments needed for mastoidectomy include: rongeur, Proud fascia crusher, House endaural retractor, endaural curettes, Jordan Day drill, and Wullstein drill with burrs. REF. 20, pp. 593, 594

442. (C) Simple mastoidectomy, removal of the air cells of the mastoid process without disturbing the contents of the middle ear, is an uncommon procedure because of the effectiveness of antibiotics in the treatment of ear infections. However, it is still the treatment of choice in the presence of complications following acute mastoiditis. REF. 20, p. 607

443. (B, C) To restore both cosmetic appearance and function, a septoplasty and rhinoplasty may be performed together. REF. 2, p. 418

444. (A, B, C) Septoplasty, septal reconstruction, and submucous resection are procedures to correct a deviated nasal septum. These names are used interchangeably. REF. 2, p. 418

445. (E) Tracheotomy, creation of a temporary or permanent opening in the trachea, requires the use of a tracheotomy tube, available in a variety of styles and sizes. Tubes must be available before the trachea is incised and ventilation control is lost. Also, the attached cuff must be tested for air leakage with a 10 cc syringe. REF. 16, pp. 348, 350

446. (A) Performance of the tracheotomy is often an emergency procedure to restore an airway and would not necessitate biopsy forceps. REF. 16, pp. 348-350

447. (A,B) The parathyroidectomy involves meticulous dissection and careful hemostasis. Identification and evaluation of four glands is required. Incision of deep cervical fascia and division of neck muscles allows exposure of the thyroid gland. REF. 23, pp. 429, 430

448. (A,B) One of the first applications of the laser was removal of laryngeal polyps. Hemostasis and simultaneous cauterization provided by the laser are advantageous working in highly vascular areas. Laser equipment has many models, accessories, and applications and is costly. Safety precautions must be taken because the laser beam is a potential igniter of any flammable material. REF. 10, pp. 11-21

449. (E) Laser safety precautions include protecting the eyes of OR personnel and patients. Wrapping the endotracheal tube and using moist patties through the laryngoscope protect the endotracheal tube against combustion and damage of the endotracheal balloon. REF. 31, pp. 6, 7

450. (A) The Hall mocro-ototome is a microdrill used in ear surgery. REF. 20, p. 602

451. (A, B, C) Tympanoplasty, repair of the tympanic membrane for patients with conductive hearing loss, may be accomplished by use of a vein graft, a fascial graft taken from the temporalis muscle behind the ear, or prosthetic substitution. REF. 20, pp. 608-609

452. (E) With the aid of the microscope, a myringotomy or incision of the tympanic membrane is done to treat acute otitis media. Following release of pus or fluid in the middle ear, hearing may be restored and infection

controlled. Tubes may be inserted through the tympanic membrane. REF. 20, p. 603

453. (A,B,D) Stapedectomy is performed to restore hearing in patients with conductive deafness. With the aid of the microscope the stapes is removed and a linkage between the incus and oval window is reestablished. A vein graft, polyethylene tube, or other prosthetic material may be used. REF. 20, p. 610

454. (A,B,C) Surgery within the eye or intraocular procedures would include cataract extraction, scleral buckling, or removal of pterygium, the fleshy triangular encroachment onto the cornea. Ectropian repair, entropian repair, and ptosis repair are extraocular procedures. REF. 2, pp. 401, 402

455. (B,E) Circular excision or trephination of the cornea is performed on both donor and recipient eyes in the corneal transplant procedure. Suturing of the donor cornea and protection of the operative eye with eye pad and Fox shield complete the procedure. REF. 16, pp. 446, 447

456. (B,C,D) Clipping the eyelashes and povidone eye preparation are the initial steps in the scleral buckling procedure. Incision of the conjunctiva, exposure of the sclera, and isolation of recti muscles are followed by creation of the chorioretinal scar with diathermy. Implants are rinsed in saline before use. REF. 30, pp. 502, 503

457. (A,B) With proper consent, eye bank specimens are removed immediately after death under aseptic conditions. Eyes are supported by a saline-soaked sponge in a sterile specimen container with the cornea up. REF. 20, p. 681

458. (C,E) The phacoemulsifier permits extracapsular cataract extraction through a very small incision. Ultrasonic vibration, irrigation, and aspiration accomplish this procedure, which has a short convalescence. REF. 2, p. 405

459. (A,B,E) Vitrectomy, removal of a portion of vitreous humor, is performed for vitreal opacities, vitreal hemorrhage, and certain types of retinal detachment. REF. 2, p. 408

460. (A, B, D) Laser delivery system employs the binocular microscope of the slip lamp, thus giving steropsis and greater magnification. The laser produces a more sharply defined burn. REF. 2, p. 407

461. (E) The IOL implant after cataract extraction allows the patient almost immediate postoperative vision. Preparation at the time of incision includes neutralization of the lens. REF. 16, pp. 453, 454

462. (B, C, D) The cryoextractor is used for lens extraction. REF. 16, pp. 454, 455

463. (A) Strabismus (squint) results from misalignment of extraocular muscles, preventing eyes from remaining in simultaneous focus on a viewed object. Surgical treatment is resection, removal of a portion of muscle and attachment of cut ends and recession; or severance of the muscle from its original insertion and reattachment more posteriorly on the sclera. REF. 20, p. 672

464. (A, B, C) Instruments included for eye muscle operations are lid speculum, muscle hooks, caliper, Steven scissors, and Castroviejo forceps and needle holder. REF. 20, p. 74

465. (C, D) Cataract extraction may be intracapsular, removing the lens within its capsule, or the more preferred extracapsular method whereby the anterior portion of the capsule is first ruptured and removed, and the lens cortex and nucleus are expressed from the eye, leaving the posterior capsule behind. Bipolar cautery is required which provides maximum cauterization with minimum tissue necrosis. REF. 20, pp. 682-687

466. (B, C) Iridectomy for treatment of glaucoma is performed to reestablish communication between the posterior and anterior chambers, thus allowing outflow of aqueous fluid through the canal of Schlemm. REF. 20, p. 688

467. (A, C, D) Scleral buckling, surgery to treat retinal detachment, causes an intrusion into the eye at the site of detachment. In addition, diathermy or cryotherapy may be used, causing an inflammatory reaction that leads to permanent adhesion between the detached retina and underlying structures. REF. 20, p. 691

468. (E) The split-thickness (partial thickness) skin grafts or full-thickness skin grafts are segments of epidermis and dermis completely separated from their blood supply before being transplanted to another area of the body. A flap is also tissue completely detached from its donor site but after transfer includes microvascular anastomoses of at least one artery and two veins (between flap and recipient site) to provide tissue viability. Compound tissues that are completely separated from blood supply of the donor site and transplanted to another area of the body are known as composite grafts. REF. 20, p. 543

469. (E) Pedical flaps are raised from the donor site with sharp dissection but not immediately severed free. The flap is sutured to the recipient site and released from the donor site when acquired vascularization has taken place, usually in 2-3 weeks. REF. 16, p. 484

470. (A, C, D) Examples of plastic/reconstructive surgery are: dermabrasion, sanding or planing of the skin to smooth scars and surface irregularities; rhinoplasty, reshaping and/or reduction in size of the nose; and blepharoplasty, removal of loose skin and protruding periorbital fat of the eylids. REF. 20, pp. 566-570

471. (B, C, D) Cleft lip is a congenital deformity, resulting in a splitting of the lip. To correct the deformity, incisions are made in the lip to allow approximation in a cosmetically appealing manner. REF. 16, pp. 499, 500

472. (B, C, D) Cleft palate creates a fissure through the roof of the mouth when tissues of the palate fail to fuse. This congenital anomaly is corrected by palatoplasty, or closure of the palate, between 18 and 24 months of age in hopes of avoiding speech defects. REF. 2, p. 470

473. (B, C, D) Rhytidectomy or facelift is excision of redundant skin of the face and upper neck resulting from the aging process. This procedure can be performed under general or local anesthesia and involves incision and undermining of the skin. REF. 20, pp. 569-571

474. (E) The use of a skin graft or skin flap for cover depends on the size and location of the defect, the blood supply, and the quality of the skin surrounding the defect. REF. 24, p. 1174

475. (D) Sterile wooden applicators and dye such as methylene blue could be substituted for sterile marking pens. REF. 16, pp. 479, 480

476. (A,B) Dermabrasion, sanding or planing of the skin, is used to smooth scars and surface irregularities of the skin. It can also be used to remove tattoos. REF. 20, p. 570

477. (D) The Erich or Jelenko splint is a method of fixation in fractures of the mandible and maxilla. Wires, lugs, and rubber bands are used to hold the teeth in occlusion. REF. 2, p. 450

478. (C,D) Brown and Hall dermatomes are oscillating blade types with adjustable depth gauges. They may be electrical or air powered. The length of the graft obtained by these instruments is limited only by the donor site. REF. 2, p. 446

479. (A, B, E) Stent fixation is used in areas where bandages cannot be applied snugly. Examples are a mold taped over the nose and long suture ends tied crisscross over a dressing. REF. 2, p. 445

480. (C,D) The latissimus dorsi myocutaneous island flap with silicone implant is a method of breast reconstruction after mastectomy. The nipple-areola area may also be reconstructed. This reconstruction does not interfere with biopsies or x-rays to detect recurrences. Chemotherapy and/or radiation therapy may delay this procedure. REF. 26, pp. 612-617

481. (B,C) Reduction mammoplasty reduces hyperplasia of the breast and involves reconstruction of breast contour, shape, and symmetry. Ptosis and back pain from poor posture and weight of breasts are indications for this procedure. REF. 20, pp. 548, 549

482. (C, D) A radical vulvectomy and groin lymphadenectomy is performed for extensive malignant disease of the vulva. It involves dissection of skin from the abdomen and groin, labia majora and minora, clitoris, mons veneris and portions of the urethra, vagina, superficial and/or deep inguinal nodes, portions of the round ligaments, portions of the saphenous veins, and the lesion itself. REF. 20, p. 317

483. (E) Vaginal repair operations or anterior/posterior repair may be performed to correct: cystocele, herniation of the bladder; rectocele, protrusion of the anterior rectal wall into the vagina; or enterocele, a herniation of cul-de-sac of Douglas. REF. 38, pp. 1703, 1704

484. (B,C) Multiple myomectomy or removal of benign symptomatic leiomyomas is a useful surgical procedure for young women with this condition who desire to bear children. REF. 38, p. 1709

485. (A,C,D) Pelvic exenteration, a radical procedure for invasive carcinoma, is not performed for palliation but when there is a possibility of a cure. Exenterations may be anterior, posterior, or complete. Reproductive organs, bladder, perineum, rectum, and pelvic lymph nodes may be involved in these procedures, depending on the extent and/or location of malignancy. REF. 2, p. 348

486. (A,B,C) Treatment of ectopic pregnancy consists of removal of the affected tube. Removal of the ovary depends on the extent of damage. REF. 2, p. 348

487. (A) The Marshall-Marchetti operation or vesicourethral suspension is an abdominal operation for correction of stress incontinence. REF. 2, p. 349

488. (E) The laparoscopy procedure provides endoscopic visualization of the peritoneal cavity through the anterior abdominal wall after establishment of a pneumoperitoneum. REF. 20, p. 333

489. (A) Carbon dioxide is slowly introduced into the peritoneal cavity via the Verres needle to create a pneumoperitoneum for laparoscopy procedure. REF. 2, p. 341

490. (A,B,D) Bandage scissors, bulb syringe, Pennington clamps, suction, bovie, and delivery forceps would be added to the abdominal gynecological instrumentation to perform a cesarean section. REF. 20, p. 346

491. (C) Closure of a cavity within a cavity (uterus) would require an additional sponge count. REF. 20, p. 34

492. (C,D) Suction curettage may be performed for missed and incomplete abortions or termination of early pregnancy.

There is less chance of uterine perforation with this procedure. REF. 20, p. 326

493. (B,C) Jackson retractors are exposing instruments for dilatation and currettage. The Gaylor biopsy forcep is used to take multiple biopsies of the cervix. REF. 20, p. 326

494. (A,D) The Shirodkar operation, placing suture at the level of the internal os, is performed to prevent cervical dilatation that results in spontaneous abortion. Endometrial or cervical insertion of cesium is for treatment of malignancy. REF. 20, pp. 328, 329

495. (A, B, C) Uterine suspension, shortening and repositioning of the uterine ligaments, may be performed in instances of pelvic inflammatory disease, endometriosis, tuboplasty, or for symptoms of uterine retroversion. REF. 20, p. 342

496. (B,C,D) Microsurgical technique is used for tubal ligation reversal. Ligation may have been performed through the laparoscope with clips, rings, or cautery. REF. 15, pp. 199-204

497. (E) Bleeding from uterine vessels must be carefully guarded against during division of broad ligaments and incision into the vagina. Other hazards of hysterectomy are injury to the bladder wall, ureters, and bowels. REF. 23, p. 363

498. (B) During the cesarean section, suction is imperative once the uterus is opened and the presenting membranes are incised. REF. 20, p. 345

499. (E) The cystoscope allows endoscopic examination of the lower urinary tract, including the urethra, bladder, ureteral orifices. The cystoscope may be a concave or convex sheath with obturator. Other accessory items for the cystoscopy procedure include various operating and catheterizing telescopes and connections for cautery equipment. REF. 20, p. 247-251

500. (A,C,D) Urethral catheters, plain and self-retaining, may be used for drainage, diagnostic studies, or stents. Some common types are Foley, Davis female urethrographic, or Robinson catheter. Malecot or Pezzer

catheters may be used to drain the bladder suprapubically. REF. 20, pp. 244-246

501. (B,C,E) Instruments needed for nephrectomy include rib shears and elevators in case a rib must be taken in order to gain access to the retroperitoneal space. Right-angle clamps or Mixters and kidney pedicle clamps are used to dissect the vessels and ureter. REF. 16, pp. 276-277

502. (C,D,E) Cystometry involves infusing fluid through a urethral or suprapubic catheter and recording pressure response. Bladder capacity and voiding pressure may be noted. REF. 38, p. 1726

503. (E) The Y-V Foley type pyeloureteroplasty is a combined correction of a redundant renal pelvis and resection of a stenotic portion of the ureteropelvic junction. The instrument set-up for this procedure includes that for nephrectomy, plus fine instruments (mosquitoes, Schnidt gall duct forceps, and fine scissors). REF. 20, p. 292

504. (E) The recipient set-up for the kidney transplant procedure includes laparotomy and vascular instruments, clip applicators, Harrington retractors, and accessory items, which include a pediatric feeding tube to be passed through the ureteroneocystostomy. REF. 20, pp. 303, 304

505. (A,B,C) Patients undergoing chronic dialysis must have an access for this procedure. This may be an external arteriovenous shunt (Scribner), a subcutaneous AV fistula, or a bovine heterograft. This procedure is most often performed under local anesthesia. REF. 2, p. 353

506. (A,B,D) The ileal conduit procedure diverts urine flow to an isolated section of bowel. One end of bowel is brought out through the skin and a stoma is created for outflow of urine. REF. 20, p. 298

507. (B,C,D) Cystectomy involves total excision of the urinary bladder and adjacent structures and requires permanent urinary diversion. It may be performed when vesical malignancy has not invaded the muscular wall of the bladder or when frequent recurrences of widespread papillary tumors do not respond to endoscopic or chemotherapeutic management. REF. 20, p. 283

508. (B,D,E) Adrenalectomy may be performed for hypersecretion of adrenal hormones, adrenal tumors, or for treatment of neoplasm elsewhere in the body that depends on adrenal hormone secretions, such as carcinoma of the prostate or breast. REF. 20, p. 299

509. (B,C) Often both adrenal glands are explored and the patient may be placed in the prone position, modified Kraske, or supine if an abdominal approach is preferred. REF. 20, p. 299

510. (A,C,D) Enlargement of the prostate gland can cause urinary obstruction. Prostatic hypertrophy may be benign or malignant. REF. 2, p. 359

511. (B,C,E) Prostatic enucleator, prostatic lobe forceps, urethral sound, Heaney needle holder, Lowsley tractors, and special retractors may be required for open prostatectomy. REF. 20, p. 275

512. (E) The retropubic approach for prostatectomy is most common because of ideal exposure and hemostasis; the suprapubic approach allows access to surgical correction of existing bladder conditions. The perineal approach may be used when open prostatic biopsy is desired. The transurethral approach may be acceptable, depending on the size of the gland, age and condition of the patient, and the presence of associated disease. REF. 20, p. 252

513. (C,D) Vasovasostomy or recannulization of the vas to restore fertility requires precise anastomosis with the aid of the operating microscope. REF. 2, p. 359

514. (A,C,D) Bilateral orchiectomy is usually performed to alter hormone secretion in patients with prostatic cancer and renders the patient sterile. Unilateral orchiectomy does not sterilize the patient and may be performed to remove a testicular tumor or may be indicated following trauma or infection. REF. 2, p. 358

515. (E) The surgical procedure to treat impotence may be insertion of the Scott inflatable prosthesis or the rigid, small carrion type. REF. 2, p. 360

516. (C,D,E) Coagulum pyeleolithotomy is a method of removing multiple small calculi from the renal collecting

system. The coagulum mixture injected into the renal pelvis forms a clot, trapping the small stones. Clot and stones are then removed. The lateral approach to the kidney is used and an intraoperative pyelogram is necessary. REF. 12, pp. 680, 684, 685

517. (E) Hemodialysis may be accomplished via venous catheterization, creation of an arteriovenous fistula, use of shunts, or placement of bovine or polytetrafluorethylene grafts. REF. 17, pp. 704, 706, 708, 710

518. (C, D, E) Hydrocelectomy is performed in the supine position through a scrotal incision. Moist sponges should be used around the wound to prevent painful postoperative swelling. REF. 23, pp. 371, 372

519. (A, B, C) Renal arteriography, cystoscopy, retrograde pyelography, and CT scan may identify the presence of a renal mass causing hematuria. Hematological studies should be carried out if there is difficulty determining the cause of hematuria. REF. 23, pp. 373, 374

520. (E) The donor nephrectomy procedure for kidney transplant requires set-up of a perfusion table, which would include cold saline and electrolyte solution, sterile IV tubing, and a venous catheter to facilitate flushing and cooling of the kidney. Forceps, scissors, and mosquitoes must be available to trim vessels and insert the catheter for flushing. REF. 20, pp. 300, 301

521. (C) A curved lower quadrant or long inguinal incision is made to facilitate placement of the kidney in the iliac fossa. REF. 16, p. 278

522. (A, B, C) The ileal loop urinary diversion connects the ureters to a conduit formed from a section of the terminal ileum. The ileum is brought to the skin to form a stoma. RE Removal of the bladder is usually the second stage of the procedure. REF. 4, pp. 712, 716, 720, 722

523. (C, D) A bottle system or compact disposable unit may be connected to chest tubes to facilitate postoperative drainage of fluid from the intrapleural or mediastinal space and to establish negative pressure in the intrapleural space. REF. 20, p. 356

524. (A,C,D,E) Instruments included for thoracic surgery would be bone instruments, Alexander, Doyen; Finochietto retractors; and the Baily rib contractor, in addition to basic and vascular instruments. REF. 20, pp. 357-360

525. (A,C) Surgical procedures involving removal of lung tissue include open lung biopsy, segmental resection, wedge resection, lobectomy, and pneumonectomy. REF. 20, pp. 370-374

526. (B,C) Thoracoplasty involves resection of ribs to obliterate the pleural cavity or to reduce thoracic space. Inadequate expansion of the lung, persistent shift of the mediastinum after pneumonectomy, or chronic empyema may be indications for this procedure. REF. 2, p. 387

527. (A,B,E) The thoracic set-up may include instruments such as Nelson and Potts scissors; Rumel, Duval and Semb forceps; various vascular instruments; and bone instruments such as Overholt elevators. REF. 20, p. 358

528. (E) Sternal and/or multiple rib fractures often produce an unstable chest wall. Internal stabilization is by controlled respiration (through tracheotomy tube). A wire or pin may be inserted through rib or sternal fragments to correct depression after elevation of the bone. Maintenance of elevation is by traction. REF. 2, p. 388

529. (A,B,C) Bronchoscopy allows direct visualization of the respiratory tree and lungs. Specimens obtained via the bronchoscope may be in the form of washings, brushings, and biopsy. REF. 16, pp. 345, 346

530. (A,B) Principles of good positioning include provision for adequate exposure and efficient ventilation and circulation. Abrupt changes in position may cause hypotension. The lateral position gives access to both the anterior and posterior surfaces of the lung. REF. 20, p. 355

531. (C) Pneumonectomy is removal of the entire lung. REF. 20, p. 374

532. (C) Esophagoscopy is direct visualization of the esophagus and the cardia of the stomach and removal of tissue or secretions for study. REF. 20, p. 369

533. (A,B,C) Collection of bronchial washings requires attachment to the suction of a container or tube designed for this purpose. The specimen container must be held in the upright position. Saline may be injected through the bronchoscope for irrigation. REF. 20, p. 368

534. (A,B) Mediastinoscopy, direct visualization of lymph nodes or tumors in the mediastinum, requires a small incision above the suprasternal notch. General anesthesia is used. If nodes are positive, treatment may be radiation or chemotherapy. REF. 20, p. 370

535. (D) The Bailey rib contractor and interrupted chromic gut sutures are used to reapproximate the ribs. REF. 20, p. 360

536. (A,C,D) The thoracic stapling instrument may be used to suture the bronchus and pulmonary vessels or applied along the limits of lung tissue to be excised in a wedge resection. REF. 20, pp. 371, 373

537. (C,D,E) Nodes that receive lymphatic drainage from the lungs and can be examined via mediastinoscopy are the subcarinal or bifurcation nodes, the superior tracheobronchial, and the paratracheal. REF. 21, pp. 59, 60

538. (E) Patients undergoing heart surgery are placed on an OR bed with a thermia blanket to control body temperature as necessary throughout the procedure. Pressure monitoring during this surgery usually includes arterial, venous, and left atrial. Extracorporeal perfusion is accomplished via the pump-oxygenator. REF. 20, p. 384

539. (E) Cardiovascular instruments include: Satinsky vena cava clamp, Harken auricle clamps, Craaford coarctation clamps, and Potts forceps, scissors, and clamps. REF. 20, p. 389

540. (B,C,D) Cardiac catheterization is insertion of a radiopaque catheter into the right or left side of the heart via a percutaneous puncture or cutdown in a peripheral vessel. The brachial or femoral vessels may be used. Sterile technique must be adhered to for this procedure. REF. 38, pp. 2174, 2183

541. (A,B) Pericardectomy involves excision of adhered, thickened fibrotic pericardium to relieve constriction of

compressed heart and large blood vessels. The pericardium is commonly exposed via a median sternotomy, although a left anterior thoracotomy with extension across the sternum into the right chest has been advocated. REF. 38, p. 2171

542. (A, B, C) A sternotomy is a midline chest incision through the sternum. Splitting of the sternum may be accomplished by use of a sternal saw blade or Lebshe sternal knife. REF. 16, p. 365

543. (E) Application of sterile talcum powder to pleural surfaces is done to stimulate growth of adhesions between the pleurae. Considerations for this procedure are recurrent spontaneous pneumothorax or palliation of excessive pleural effusions related to inoperable malignancies. REF. 20, p. 375

544. (C, D) Ventricular septal defect is one of the most common congenital cardiac anomalies. If small, a murmur is evident, but other symptoms may not be present. A larger murmur producing enlarged heart and left-to-right shunt requires surgery. REF. 38, pp. 2254-2256

545. (A, B, C) Electrodes for permanent cardiac pacing may be placed via the transthoracic method or the transvenous method. The transvenous (endocardiac) is preferred because thoracotomy and general anesthesia are not required. Also, an alternate technique of placing myocardial electrodes may be performed through a subxiphoid incision. REF. 20, pp. 421-423

546. (B) Atherosclerosis is most frequently the cause of occlusive disease of the major branches of the aorta. Arterial sites more susceptible to stenosis or occlusion are at the origins of vessels where turbulence may be present. REF. 38, p. 1921

547. (B, D) Arterial injuries should be repaired within the first 4 hr after injury. Repair may involve control of bleeding by application of vascular clamps, resection of damaged vessel, and end-to-end anastomosis. Synthetic or venous grafts may also be required. REF. 38, pp. 1969, 1970

548. (A) An endarterectomy involves surgical removal of intraluminal atheromatous obstructive plaques. REF. 20, p. 430

549. (E) Pulmonary embolism may be a complication of surgery and originate from veins in the lower extremities. Treatment may include vena cava clipping or a filter procedure for partial vena cava occlusion on poor-risk patients. REF. 2, pp. 392, 398

550. (C) Localized abnormal dilation of an artery with formation of a sac, caused by pressure of blood on the weakened wall, is an aneurysm. REF. 2, p. 397

551. (E) Dissecting aneurysms occur following degeneration of the medial layer of the vessel. A combination of factors leads to an intimal tear followed by the development of a dissecting hematoma into the media of the vessel wall. REF. 38, p. 1877

552. (A,C,D) Acute aortic dissection is usually not limited to the ascending aorta or aortic arch. REF. 38, p. 1877

553. (A,C) Various shunt procedures between the hypertensive portal and lower caval circulation result in lowering portal pressure with disappearance of varices and protection against hemorrhage. Manometer, stopcock, P-E tubing, syringe, and needles should be included in the set-up for this operation to measure portal pressures. REF. 20, p. 440

554. (E) To facilitate hemodialysis, arteriovenous shunts may be performed. This procedure would require a minor instrument set plus vascular instruments (bulldogs, forceps, Potts scissors, arterial dilators) and vessel appliances. Saline and heparin solution are necessary for irrigation. REF. 20, p. 442

555. (A,B,E) If anticoagulant therapy fails, ligation of the vena cava may be performed to prevent pulmonary embolism. This may be accomplished by suture ligation or application of a Teflon clip which allows partial flow of venous blood to reduce vascular congestion in the lower extremities. REF. 20, pp. 442, 443

556. (C) A balloon catheter provides a safe, effective means to extract arterial emboli. REF. 38, p. 1977

557. (A,B,C) Vascular grafts can be venous autographs, arterial allographs, modified bovine grafts (arterial xenograph), or textile prosthetic grafts. REF. 38, pp. 1864-1866

558. (E) Coronary surgery requires sternotomy incision and harvesting of the saphenous vein to be used for the bypass vein graft. Extracorporeal circulation or cardiopulmonary bypass and moderate hypothermia are necessary for this procedure. REF. 20, p. 402

559. (E) The purpose of the pump oxygenator used during open heart surgery is to circulate, cool, filter, oxygenate, and perfuse the blood to vital organs. REF. 23, p. 468

560. (C,D) Cannulae are inserted into the vena cava and ascending aorta in order that pump tubing may be connected to collect, oxygenate, and return blood to the body. Occasionally the femoral artery and vein are used. REF. 16, p. 367

561. (B) The coronary artery bypass operation uses an autologous vein graft to bypass an occluded segment of one or more coronary arteries. REF. 16, p. 377

562. (A,D) Prosthetic heart valves are mechanical or biological. Mechanical are ball and cage, or tilting disc valve. Biological valves include the porcine bioprosthesis and the bovine pericardial xenograft. REF. 40, pp. 965, 966

563. (E) Survival of the increasing number of heart transplant patients has improved with the possibility of distant heart procurement, improved immunosuppression, and early detection of rejection and infection. REF. 28, pp. 45, 481

564. (A,C) An alternative to replacing the mitral valve might be the mitral commissurotomy, or opening of the commissures that bring the cusps of the valve together. Also, sutures in the annulus (mitral annuloplasty) may allow the valve leaflets to come together more efficiently. REF. 16, p. 385

565. (D, E) Valve instruments and prosthetic graft would be needed for resection of ascending aortic aneurysm. REF. 16, p. 385

566. (B) Passage of a balloon tip catheter into the narrowed coronary artery with subsequent cautious inflation to slightly dilate the vessel and compress the plaque is angioplasty. If successful, it is an alternative to coronary artery bypass surgery. REF. 36, p. 199

567. (B, C, D) Transthoracic and transvenous are the two methods of placing electrodes for permanent cardiac pacing. The transthoracic approach would require an anterolateral thoracotomy. REF. 20, p. 422

568. (E) Carotid endarterectomy requires clamping of the internal, external, and common carotid arteries. Temporary bypass may be used. Blunt dissectors and Potts scissors facilitate plaque removal. A patch angioplasty may be necessary. REF. 20, pp. 434, 435

569. (C) A common injury to the wrist is the carposcaphoid fracture. REF. 38, p. 1544

570. (B) The Colles' fracture of the distal forearm is transverse with dorsal and radial displacement. REF. 38, p. 1542

571. (A, D, E) Bennett retractors, Loman holding clamp, and Creggo elevators would be added to the basic bone instrument set for fixation of intertrochanteric fractures. REF. 20, p. 491

572. (E) Occasionally, knee joint operations may require the knee flexed. Instruments specifically designed for knee operations are necessary. Bone grafts or metal prostheses may be employed. REF. 20, p. 519

573. (A, B, C) Treatment of bone infection, osteomyelitis, may require surgery, debridement of bone and soft tissue, removal of nonviable bone, and insertion of catheters for instillation of antibiotics. REF. 38, p. 1599

574. (C) Arthroscopy provides visualization via the arthroscope of the knee joint and can aid in diagnosis of knee

disorders. Arthrotomy, or incision into the joint, may be necessary to perform a biopsy, remove cartilage, or repair defects. REF. 2, p. 375

575. (D) The development of the total hip arthroplasty has replaced procedures such as subtrochanteric osteotomy, cup arthroplasty, and prosthetic head replacement in nearly all instances of hip reconstruction. REF. 20, p. 500

576. (A, B, C) Patellectomy set-up requires regular bone and soft tissue instruments, knee instruments, drill and bits, and heavy wire. REF. 20, pp. 509, 511

577. (B, D) Elevation of the articular surface following central depression fracture of the tibial plateau may be accomplished through a window in the anterior tibia packed with bone to give additional support. REF. 20, p. 510

578. (A, B) The treatment of choice for osteosarcoma is amputation. Chemotherapy and radiotherapy may be combined or used alone in treatment of unresectable tumors or in the presence of metastatic disease. REF. 14, p. 67

579. (A, B) Meticulous aseptic technique is critical in orthopedic surgery because infection in bone can remain for life or result in loss of an extremity. Orthopedic operations are often performed in contaminated tissue or tissues highly susceptible to infection. REF. 2, p. 367

580. (B, C, D) Orthopedic instruments require special care and handling, such as sharpening of cutting instruments, e.g., chisels, gouges. Each instrument has a specific purpose and is not interchangeable. Implant-related instruments, cutting instruments, and exposing instruments are examples of categories of orthopedic instruments by design. REF. 2, p. 367

581. (C) Bone wax may be used for hemostasis in bone. REF. 2, p. 369

582. (B) The type of suture preferred for periosteum is usually absorbable. REF. 2, p. 370

583. (A, B, D) Ligaments, tendons, and muscles involved in movements of bony structures are usually sutured with nonabsorbable materials. REF. 2, p. 371

584. (D) Casts should be cut and removed before patients are transferred to the OR because plaster dust causes airborne contamination of the sterile tables with plaster dust. REF. 2, p. 370

585. (C, E) Knowledge of and special preparation of the orthopedic table are important for proper use of this equipment. The circo-electric bed is often used postoperatively after spinal procedures. REF. 20, p. 459

586. (C, D) Imperfections are inevitable with the use of implantation devices. The strength of an implant may be affected by scratches, abrasions, and similar damage. REF. 20, p. 461

587. (E) Orthopedic instruments, supplies, and equipment require special handling, storage, and sterilization to prevent alteration in strength, composition, and surface. REF. 20, p. 461

588. (B) An OR table which permits 90° flexion of the knee should be used for arthroscopy. REF. 6, p. 10

589. (D) The Bankart procedure is one operation designed to strengthen the anterior joint capsule of the shoulder. REF. 20, pp. 476, 477

590. (A, C, D, E) Bronchoscopy, esophagoscopy, and mediastinoscopy are endoscopic procedures pertinent to thoracic surgery. Topical or general anesthetic may be used. Topical anesthetic set-up includes sprays, laryngeal mirrors, Jackson forceps, and various medications. REF. 20, p. 361

591. (A, B) Lymphangiography is used to visualize lymphatic vessels and interconnecting lymph nodes. This procedure is accomplished by injection of contrast material via a fine catheter within a lymphatic by use of an infusion pump. REF. 38, pp. 1794, 1795

592. (A, C) Fiberoptic urological instruments are delicate and complex and therefore require OR personnel well versed in the care and handling of these instruments. This equipment differs from other fiberoptic instruments in that they are rigid and have various telescopes to provide different angle views of the urological system. REF. 16, pp. 294, 295

593. (E) Colonoscopy is a widely accepted procedure to diagnose and treat some lesions of the colon and rectum. REF. 13, p. 45

594. (D) Gastroscopy may be performed to evaluate an upper GI bleed and to determine the benign or malignant nature of a lesion. Pre- and postoperative evaluation of candidates for partial gastrectomy may be accomplished by use of the gastroscope. Also, direct visualization of gastric or duodenal ulcers may determine the specific choice of therapy, conservative or surgical. REF. 13, p. 47

595. (A,C,D) Initial steps in the craniotomy procedure require the use of angled Weitlaner retractors once the incision has been made. The pericranium is stripped with a periosteal elevator and burr holes may be made with a perforator or craniotome. Gigli saws and guide or air drill may be used to cut between the burr holes. REF. 16, p. 429

596. (B) Wet, compressed rayon-cotton pledgets (cottonoid) are used during brain and spinal cord surgery. Coarse-gauge sponges will injure these fragile tissues. REF. 16, p. 430

597. (E) Exposing instruments for neurosurgical procedures require various self-retaining retractors (Weitlaners, Gelpi, mastoid) and several types of periosteal elevators. REF. 20, p. 732

598. (A,B,D) CAT scan produces cross-sectional x-rays of the brain or other areas of the body. Ventricles of the brain, blood vessels, tumors, and other structures are represented in pictorial x-rays. REF. 16, p. 422

599. (A,C,E) Instrumentation for craniotomy includes the basic set plus general and specific instruments preferred by the operating surgeon. The basic dissecting kit would include several types of forceps including bayonet and Cushing, spatulas, and assorted retractors including malleables. REF. 20, p. 733

600. (B,C) Operation for the acute subdural hematoma depends on the consistency of the clot. If liquid, multiple trephinations and a small temporal craniectomy are required. If a solid clot is encountered, a temporoparietal skull flap is required. REF. 38, p. 1487

601. (E) Percutaneous cordotomy is considered a blind operation usually reserved for poor-risk patients. This procedure is performed under local anesthesia with roentgenographic control of a coagulating needle guided into the anterolateral quadrant of the spinal cord. REF. 38, p. 1512

602. (A,B,D) An intracranial aneurysm can cause fatal hemorrhage, which is often the first symptom. To prevent this, control of blood pressure as well as the vascular supply to the region beyond the limits of the lesion may be required. REF. 20, pp. 743, 744

603. (B,D,E) Most intracranial aneurysms are associated with a congenital defect of the media of the intracranial tissue wall. Enlargement, outpouching, and thinning of the arterial wall eventually leads to rupture. An aneurysm may impinge on the third nerve or the optic chiasm. REFS. 20, p. 743; 2, p. 436

604. (A,C) Peripheral neurectomies of the supraorbital or infraorbital nerves to treat trigeminal neuralgia may be temporary because the nerves regenerate. Retrogasserian neurectomy by a temporal or posterior fossa approach or retrogasserian rhizotomy with radiofrequency current are more certain methods of obtaining relief. REF. 20, p. 710

605. (A,C,D) A basic neurosurgical instrument set plus special laminectomy instruments are needed for surgery of the vertebrae. Spurling-Kerrison rongeurs, Beckman-Adson and Adson self-retaining retractors, Horsley bone cutter, and Scoville retractors are some of these. REF. 20, p. 765

606. (B,C,E) Laminectomy, removal of one or more vertebral laminae, may be performed to treat compression fractures, dislocations, herniated discs, or cord tumor or for insertion of subarachnoid shunts. REF. 20, p. 764

607. (A,D) Injury to motor roots resulting in paralysis and bleeding from epidural veins, which is difficult to control, are the most significant hazards of vertebral and spinal cord surgery. REF. 23, p. 488

608. (A,C) Sympathectomy procedure is often done to relieve arterial spasm of vascular disease, to increase vascular

circulation, or to treat intractable pain of advanced carcinoma. Various locations along the spinal column may be approached. A flank incision or transperitoneal paramedian incision may be preferred. REF. 16, p. 423

609. (C,D) Carpal tunnel release, incision or excision of the transverse carpal ligament with or without synovectomy within the canal, may be performed to relieve symptoms caused by compression of the median nerve. REF. 20, p. 583

610. (A,B,E) Laminectomy, removal of one or more vertebrae to expose the spinal cord, is often performed for herniated disc. The level of the spinal column to be operated on determines if the patient will be in lateral, prone, or sitting position. Basic neurosurgery, cautery, and laminectomy instruments are necessary for this procedure. REF. 22, p. 388

611. (A,B) Bipolar cautery forceps isolate current output completely between the forcep tips, thus causing less tissue damage. A grounding pad is not required. REF. 22, p. 389

612. (C,E) Pituitary rongeurs of various sizes and angles can be used to remove herniated disc material, to remove tumor, or to biopsy brain tissue. REF. 22, pp. 390, 391

613. (B,C) A craniotomy is performed to expose a cerebral aneurysm. Visualization is improved with the use of the operating microscope and accessories. Treatment may be application of metallic clips or coating with plastic if clipping is not feasible. Ligation of affected vessels may be necessary if neither clipping nor coating can be done. REF. 23, p. 493

614. (B,C,D) Hair must be removed with clippers for craniotomy procedures. For the posterior fossa craniotomy, the patient would usually be placed in Fowler's or sitting position with the head supported by a headrest. When the brain is higher than the heart (sitting position), prevention of potential air embolism must be considered. A double Mayo set-up is usually preferred. REF. 2, p. 433

615. (D) The dura guard attachment for the air-powered drill protects the dura mater during craniotomy. REF. 2, p. 433

616. (B) The subarachnoid screw placed in the subarachnoid space allows attachment of continuous or intermittent pressure monitoring devices. REF. 2, p. 434

617. (A, B, D) Cerebral revascularization provides a source of blood to the cerebral circulation by anastomosis of an extracranial artery to an intracranial artery. REF. 2, pp. 435, 436

618. (E) Pituitary tumors may be removed via the transphenoidal hypophysectomy. It can also be a palliative procedure to relieve symptoms of metastatic cancer. A muscle, fat, or fascial graft may be necessary to pack the sella turcica. REF. 2, p. 436

619. (C, D) Shunting procedures, ventriculoatrial or ventriculoperitoneal, divert spinal fluid away from the brain to the atrium of the heart or to the peritoneum. REF. 16, p. 430

620. (B, C, D) Pediatric surgical procedures include the following: repair of imperforate anus, repair of esophageal atresia, and resection and pull-through of the colon for Hirschsprung's disease. REF. 20, pp. 784-799

621. (E) Hypertrophic pyloric stenosis, a common condition in infancy, obstructs emptying of the stomach. It is more common in males and involves hereditary factors. Vomiting is frequent, becomes projectile, and results in dehydration. REF. 38, p. 1379

622. (A, B, C) If the omphalocele is large, silastic sheeting may be inserted over the sac and under freed skin edges to form a protective covering. If skin edges cannot be approximated, 0.5% silver nitrate may be applied to inhibit bacterial growth. Another method is postponement of surgery and treatment of surrounding skin with mercurochrome until eschar develops, which strengthens the sac, or treatment of the sac with moist 0.5% silver nitrate dressing. REF. 20, p. 790

623. (B,C) A variety of treatment methods for neurogenic bladder may include mechanical procedures, drugs, and/or surgical procedures including urinary diversion and creation of an ileal conduit. REF. 38, p. 1759

624. (A,C,D) Except during infancy, the operation for aortic stenosis is performed with cardiopulmonary bypass. The heart is exposed via a median sternotomy incision. Risks of this operation are small and results good. REF. 38, pp. 2308, 2309

625. (B) Infants lose heat by evaporation, radiation, and conduction. Measures to prevent heat loss and hypothermia include use of warm solutions, warm blankets, and telethermometer to monitor the temperature throughout the operation. REF. 2, p. 459

626. (D) Circumcision or excision of the foreskin of the penis is a commonly performed pediatric operation to prevent phimosis. REF. 2, p. 463

627. (A, B, C) Orchipexy, surgery for undescended testicles, usually is performed at age 5 or 6. It is often a two-stage Torek orchiopexy. REF. 2, p. 463

628. (A, D) Closure of a tracheoesophageal fistula and anastomosis of the segments of the esophagus is accomplished through a right retropleural thoracotomy. REF. 20, p. 787

629. (B) A segment of colon without ganglia that results in increased tone and lack of peristalsis proximally is known as Hirschsprung's disease. REF. 20, p. 793

630. (A,B) Both Hirschsprung's disease and imperforate anus require a temporary colostomy as well as further pelvic operative procedures. REF. 20, p. 792

631. (A,B) If reduction of intussusception by the hydrostatic pressure of a barium enema is unsuccessful, then laparotomy and manual manipulation must be performed. REF. 20, p. 792

632. (C) Wilm's tumor of the kidney presents a firm, painless mass that should be entirely removed if it does not place the patient in jeopardy. REF. 20, p. 798

633. (B,D) Myringotomy with tube insertion, a common pediatric procedure, often can be performed in outpatient clinics. After proper preparation of the external ear, a slit incision is made in the eardrum and a tube inserted to reestablish full air exchange between the outer and middle ear. REF. 30, p. 626

634. (A,B,D) Essentially well children who need correction of a physical defect could have procedures such as cystoscopy, eye muscle procedures, hernia repair, and closed reduction of fractures performed on an outpatient basis. REF. 20, p. 780

635. (A, B, C) To relieve constriction of compressed heart and large blood vessels, pericardectomy or partial excision of adhered, thickened, fibrotic pericaridum may be performed. This is an acquired condition. REF. 20, p. 396

636. (B) Premature fusing of the suture lines in the skull is craniosynostosis. A craniectomy is performed to reopen the suture line and allow normal expansion of the skull. REF. 2, p. 469

637. (B) If discovered in infancy, closed reduction and immobilization may correct a congenital dislocated hip or displaced femoral head. REF. 2, p. 464

638. (E) Heat transfer to the body can be caused by flame, scalding water, electrical current, radiation, and chemicals. REF. 16, p. 511

639. (E) The first degree burn involves only the outer layer of epidermis. Redness and some pain occur, but healing is rapid. REF. 2, p. 453

640. (C,D) Burns are classified by the depth of tissue destruction that has occurred. First degree involves only the outside layer of epidermis and produces pain and reddening of the skin. Second degree burns injure the entire epidermis and a portion of the dermis; pain, blister formation, and reddish-pink, molted discoloration followed by a brown crust which separates from underlying tissues are characteristics. A third degree burn involves the entire skin thickness, is painless, and is dry and white. The burn develops a thick, black crust (eschar). There is no chance of spontaneous regeneration of epithelium with this type of burn. REF. 16, p. 511

641. (B,D,E) Extent of burn damage may be estimated by the rule of nines. The body surface of an adult is divided into areas equal to multiples of 9% of the total body surface. The head and neck equal 9%; the anterior and posterior trunks, 18% each; the upper extremities equal 9% each; the lower extremities equal 18% each; and the perineum equals 1%. REF. 2, p. 453

642. (E) The Lund and Brower chart estimates percentage of burn on the basis of age in addition to the anatomical location of the burn. REF. 2, p. 453

643. (A,B,E) Initial care of the burn patient includes removing all clothing and other objects in contact with the patient's skin. If the respiratory system is damaged, endotracheal intubation or tracheotomy may be necessary. Restoration of fluid and electrolyte balance necessitates IV therapy and placement of a retention catheter. Cleansing of the wound and estimation of extent and depth of burn are also initial considerations. REF. 2, p. 454

644. (E) Operative procedures for burn patients are many. Common ones are escharotomy, debridement, various types of skin grafts, fasciotomy, dressing changes, and amputation of digits. REF. 2, pp. 454, 455

645. (E) Environmental considerations are most important for burn patients. These may include reverse or protective isolation technique, hyperbaric oxygen, laminar airflow, and plastic isolator. Patients may be placed on Stryker frames or circo-electric beds. REF. 2, pp. 455, 456

646. (A,B) Serial biopsy cultures are taken every 2 or 3 days until the eschar of a burn begins to separate. These biopsies monitor growth of organisms and assist in determining antibiotic or chemotherapeutic agents necessary. REF. 2, p. 455

647. (B,C,E) Meshgrafts are a form of split-thickness autograft to cover large or irregular areas. Sulfadiazine cream is an antimicrobial agent common to treatment of burns. REF. 2, pp. 454, 455

648. (B) Radioactive substances are used to injure or destroy cells. Radiation is the emission of electromagnetic waves or atomic particles by disintegration of the nuclei of unstable or radioactive elements. REF. 2, p. 475

649. (C,D) Each atom of an element has the same physical and chemical properties (same number of protons). An isotope, a different form of the same element, may exist, one that has the same number of protons but a different number of neutrons. With the use of nuclear reactors and high-speed particle accelerators, it is possible to bombard a stable isotope with additional free neutrons, thus forming an unstable or radioactive isotope. REF. 8, pp. 247, 248

650. (E) Cancer is considered a group of distinct diseases with varied causes, manifestations, treatments, and prognoses. Cancer cells are abnormal cells formed from normal cells by some poorly understood mechanism of change. As this abnormal or disease process progresses, invasive properties develop and invade surrounding tissues. Then, through blood and lymph, these cells can be transported to other parts of the body (metastases). REF. 8, p. 225

651. (E) Ionizing radiation may be the primary treatment for malignancy. X-rays and gamma rays are electromagnetic radiations. A similar type of radiation is delivered by supervoltage x-ray apparatus obtained from radioisotopes cobalt 60 and cesium 137. Radioisotopes are a method of delivering ionizing radiation that is versatile and convenient to administer. Other forms are radioactive colloidal gold, interstitial needles of gold, radon, tantalum, or IV injections of sodium phosphate. REF. 8, pp. 255, 256

652. (B,C,D) Radiation therapy may cause the skin of the irradiated area to be fragile and sensitive, may prolong wound healing, and may make wound closure more difficult. Also, the cancer patient may be debilitated and malnourished. REF. 22, p. 186

653. (B) Radium is more hazardous than its substitutes because of the type of radiation rays it emits. Radium remains radioactive indefinitely and is potentially hazardous for thousands of years. REF. 22, p. 175

654. (B,D,E) The cardinal factors of protection against radiation exposure are distance, time, and shielding. REF. 2, p. 479

VI. Miscellaneous

655. (A,B) The Wertheim or radical hysterectomy procedure is removal of all recognizable lymph nodes in the pelvis and removal of the uterus, tubes, ovaries, supporting ligaments, and upper vagina. REF. 20, p. 337

656. (B) The Ramstedt-Fredet pyloromyotomy is performed to treat congenital pyloric stenosis, which is hypertrophy of the pyloric spincter obstructing the stomach. REF. 20, p. 790

657. (B,C,D) Synthetic mesh materials, such as Marlex mesh, can be used to correct congenital, traumatic, or acquired defects in fascia or a body wall and for reinforcement, as in hernia repair. REF. 2, p. 267

658. (A) A sump drain may be placed in a wound to facilitate irrigation, aspiration with suction, or introduction of medication to an area; thus it has a double or triple lumen. Lateral openings in the catheter prevent clogging. REF. 2, p. 248

659. (A, B, C) Bovine carotid artery heterographs may be used for blood access in patients on hemodialysis who have vessels inadequate for creation of fistulas or shunts. REF. 2, p. 248

660. (E) Surgical treatment for exstrophy of the bladder requires reconstruction of the lower abdominal wall, external genitalia, and provision for the passage of urine. REF. 2, p. 463

661. (D) Stapling instruments reduce the amount of tissue manipulation and handling and allow nutrition to pass through the staple line to the cut edge of the tissue. Use of these instruments decreases operating time and reduces the possibility of infection and tissue reaction. REF. 20, p. 106

662. (D) The use of Xylocaine with epinephrine enhances the length of anesthesia by causing vasoconstriction and allowing the drug to remain at the site for a longer period of time. REF. 23, p. 90

663. (E) Repair of fractures of the mandible, maxilla, and other facial fracture operations require a combination of nasal, dental, and orthopedic instruments. REF. 16, p. 503

664. (A,B,D) The most common complications of laparoscopy reported are perforation of a hollow viscus (e.g., intestine), hemorrhage from a punctured vessel or biopsy site, gas embolism, and burns of the abdominal wall and bowel. REF. 2, p. 341

665. (A,B,D) Cryosurgery provides local freezing of diseased tissue without harm to normal adjacent structures. Liquid nitrogen, carbon dioxide, or freon may be used for this procedure. REF. 2, p. 250

666. (B) Prothrombin, essential for the clotting process, is produced in liver from vitamin K. Normal prothrombic activity in the blood is dependent on adequate absorption of vitamin K from the GI tract. REF. 8, p. 503

667. (A) Usually performed to remove stretch marks and redundant fat of the lower abdomen, the abdominoplasty procedure also repairs any laxity of the rectus muscle. REF. 20, p. 572

668. (A,B,C) Outpatient surgery facilities are increasing in popularity because of escalating costs of inpatient care. Also, they can provide better utilization of hospital facilities and this service can be integrated into major OR facilities. Special concern for designing of this facility would be a one-way traffic pattern. A recovery room, observation room, or overnight room in some independent facilities would be available. REF. 20, pp. 24, 25

669. (E) Outpatients may have general or local anesthesia. OR personnel working in these areas must have special consideration for patients, as they are fully awake when they enter the facility. Outpatients often require fewer lab tests because they are healthier and require less complicated procedures. REF. 20, pp. 24, 25

670. (D) Charnley, Charnley-Muller, Bechtol, and Aufranc-Turner are names of total hip implants. REF. 20, p. 500

671. (B,C,D) Several whole pancreatic autotransplants have been performed since 1966, but the transplants are still restricted. Segmental, vascularized autotransplantation of the body and tail of the pancreas have produced promising results. REF. 38, pp. 537-542

672. (E) Multiple arterial anastomoses, biliary duct anastomosis, complexities of anesthesia management, bleeding, and failure to produce normal coagulation are all factors that contribute to the complexity of liver transplants. REF. 39, pp. 403, 405

673. (C,E) Factors that have been identified as having a direct relationship to the incidence of infection include: (1) long preoperative hospitalization; (2) lack of preoperative bathing with antiseptic solution; (3) preoperative shaving the day before surgery, (4) long operations; (5) use of electrosurgical knife; and (6) use of abdominal drains. REF. 44, pp. 9, 12-14

674. (B,D,E) Ultrasonography uses no ionizing radiation and has no side effects. This diagnostic procedure is not automated and does require great skill of the operator. Abdominal and pelvic organs can be studied and presence of cysts or solid masses can often be identified with this procedure. REF. 14, p. 88

675. (B,C) Penile implants have a high success rate of ending impotence. Insertion of the inflatable prosthesis is more complicated than the semirigid. There are advantages and disadvantages to both types that must be discussed with the patient preoperatively. REF. 33, pp. 487-494

676. (C) Storing marrow and returning it to the patient (bone marrow transplant) allows patients to receive otherwise fatal doses of chemotherapy and radiation to kill malignant cells. Patients are positioned prone, as the marrow is most commonly obtained from the posterior iliac crests. REF. 27, pp. 386, 387

677. (E) Nissen fundoplication is repair of a hiatus hernia usually performed through an upper midabdominal incision. To prevent esophogeal reflux, a fold of the fundal wall is sutured around the esophagus. Prior placement of the large lumen gastric tube ensures the plication is not too tight and aids in identification of the esophagus. REF. 41, pp. 39, 40

678. (A,C) The Broviac catheter is a long-term, indwelling catheter placed for the administration of IV fluids, chemotherapy, or antibiotics. It may be inserted through the cephalic vein to be positioned in the superior vena cava or right atrium. REF. 32, pp. 215, 216

679. (A, B, C) Surgical correction of scoliosis can involve the Harrington system. The Dywer technique may supplement this instrumentation for correction of severe spinal deformities. A body cast is applied several days postoperatively. REF. 37, pp. 42, 46

680. (A,B,C) Cardiopulmonary resuscitation must begin with establishing an airway, providing artificial ventilation, and providing artificial circulation by external cardiac compression. REF. 8, pp. 1083, 1084

681. (A, C, D) Priorities in the event of thoracic injuries would be to ensure the airway, assist with physical exam, and insert a chest tube. Unless the patient is in shock, the head and chest should be elevated. Preparation for blood transfusion is also necessary. REF. 8, p. 1092

682. (B, C, D) If there is no cervical spine injury, the patient should be positioned prone or semiprone to facilitate drainage from the tracheobronchial tree and to minimize aspiration of nasopharyngeal and gastric secretions. REF. 8, p. 1094

683. (D) Lumbar epidural block is a regional anesthesia technique for vaginal or cesarean delivery. REF. 9, pp. 263, 264

684. (E) Fetal distress occurs when maternal-fetal gas exchange is disturbed within the umbilical cord or the placenta. Maternal and/or fetal conditions such as umbilical cord problems may cause the distress. REF. 9, pp. 424, 425

685. (C) Premature separation of the placenta from the uterine wall causes bleeding that may be apparent or concealed, mild or severe. This is an obstetrical emergency requiring immediate management. REF. 9, pp. 263, 264

686. (A, B, C) Vital signs should be recorded immediately to ensure accuracy. If they are difficult to read or take, seek

assistance and alert the nurse or physician of abnormal values. REF. 16, p. 201

687. (A, B) Chest tubes must be securely attached to a sterile closed drainage system. They must always be clamped when disconnected. To prevent re-entrance of air and fluid into the chest cavity, the drainage system must be maintained at a position lower than the patient's body. REF. 20, p. 357

688. (E) Bladder catheterization requires strict aseptic technique in order to prevent bladder infection. Proper preparation of the patient and equipment are essential for performing this procedure safety and efficiently. REF. 16, pp. 201, 202

689. (B, D, E) Invasive monitoring means that a catheter is placed into a blood vessel, heart chamber, or cerebral spinal fluid space. Examples are arterial, central nervous pressure, or pulmonary artery wedge pressure monitoring. REF. 22, p. 313

690. (A, B, D) If desired results from electrocautery are not obtained, to continue increasing power is dangerous. The OR nurse and technician should check the entire system to be sure contacts with power source, pencil cable, and ground plates are complete. REF. 22, p. 358

691. (A) Pneumatic tourniquets, used in extremity surgery, restrict the venous blood flow but do not totally prevent the arterial flow. REF. 22, p. 379

REFERENCES

1. Association of Operating Room Nurses, Inc., AORN Standards of Practice for Perioperative Nursing, Denver, 1983.

2. Atkinson, L. and Kohn, M. Berry and Kohn's Introduction to Operating Room Technique, 5th ed. New York: McGraw-Hill Book Co., 1978.

3. Atkinson, L. Trends in Gastrointestinal Surgery. Ethicon/ Point of View, July 1981, pp. 4, 5.

4. Barrett, N. Ileal Loop and Body Image. AORN Journal, Oct. 1982, pp. 712, 716, 720, 722.

5. Beck, W. Hematology, 3rd ed. Cambridge: MIT Press, 1981.

6. Brown, R. Arthroscopy, A New Look in Orthopedics. JORRI, Dec. 1981, pp. 8-16.

7. Brozenec, S. Surgical Implants, Medication and Alimentation Devices. AORN Journal, June 1983, pp. 1335-1368.

8. Brunner, L. and Suddarth, D. Textbook of Medical-Surgical Nursing, 3rd ed. Philadelphia: J. B. Lippincott Co., 1975.

9. Buckley, K. and Kulb, N., (eds.). Handbook of Maternal-Newborn Nursing. Bethany, CT: Fleshner Publishing Co., 1983.

10. Burkhart, S. The Medical Use of Lasers. JORRI, April 1982, pp. 11-21.

11. Dienhart, C. M. Basic Human Anatomy and Physiology, 3rd ed. Philadelphia: W. B. Saunders Co., 1979.

12. Dillon, M. Coagulum Pyelolithotomy to Remove Multiple Stones. AORN Journal, Oct. 1982, pp. 680, 684, 688, 689.

13. Doll, L. Fiberoptics, Chapter II, State of the Art. JORRI, Jan. 1982, pp. 43-49.

14. Dumphy, J. and Way, L., (eds.). Current Surgical Diagnosis and Treatment, 5th ed. Los Altos: Lange Medical Publications, 1981.

15. Fleming, C. and Jenks, A. Microscope Tubal Reversal. AORN Journal, Feb. 1983, pp. 199-204.

16. Fuller, J. Surgical Technology, Principles and Practice. Philadelphia: W. B. Saunders Co., 1981.

17. Gould, D. Vascular Access Procedures for Hemodialysis. AORN Journal, Oct. 1982, pp. 704, 706, 708, 710.

18. Gray, J. Surviving the Survey: What to Do When JCAH is Coming. AORN Journal, June 1983, pp. 1275-1279.

19. Groah, L. Operating Room Nursing, The Perioperative Role. Reston, Va.: Reston Publishing Co., Inc., 1983.

20. Gruendemann, B. and Meeker, M. Alexander's Care of the Patient in Surgery, 7th ed. St. Louis: C. V. Mosby Co., 1983.

21. Kildea, J. Mediastinoscopy in Bronchogenic Carcinoma. AORN Journal, Jan. 1981, pp. 57-63.

22. Kneedler, J. and Dodge G. Perioperative Patient Care. Boston: Blackwell Scientific Publication, 1983.

23. LeMaitre, G. and Finnegan, J. The Patient in Surgery: A Guide for Nurses, 4th ed. Philadelphia: W. B. Saunders Co., 1980.

24. Lyons, R. Promoting Healing of Skin Flaps and Grafts. AORN Journal, May 1982, p. 1174.

25. MacCelland, D. Koch Pouch: A New Type of Ileostomy. AORN Journal, Aug. 1980, pp. 191-201.

26. Maudlin, B. Breast Reconstruction after Mastectomy. AORN Journal, March 1980, pp. 612-617.

27. Maudlin, B. Harvest of Hope: Bone Marrow Transplant. AORN Journal, Sept. 1982, pp. 385-390.

28. Miller, J. Update on Heart Transplantation. AORN Journal, July 1982, pp. 45-59.

29. Moore, C. Scleral Buckling for Retinal Detachment. AORN Journal, Sept. 1982, pp. 502, 503.

30. Moore, J. Establishment of an Outpatient ENT Clinic. AORN Journal, March 1980, pp. 620, 623, 626, 627, 630.

31. Mullaney, C. Laser Surgery in Otolaryngology. Ethicon/ Point of View, Oct. 1980, pp. 6, 7.

32. Nonkin, R. The Broviac Catheter: O. R. Technique. AORN Journal, Feb. 1982, pp. 215-217.

33. Parker, C. Ambulatory Surgery for a Penile Prosthesis. AORN Journal, Sept. 1982, pp. 487-494.

34. Physician's Desk Reference, 37th ed. Oradell, N. Y.: Medical Economics Co. Inc., 1983.

35. Phipps, W., et al. Medical Surgical Nursing. St. Louis: C. V. Mosby Co., 1979.

36. Purcell, J. Coronary Angioplasty. AORN Journal, Feb. 1982, pp. 199-206.

37. Reeder, J. Adult Scoliosis: A Personal Experience. AORN Journal, Jan. 1981, pp. 35-50.

38. Sabiston, D., (ed.). Davis-Christopher Textbook of Surgery, 12th ed. Philadelphia: W. B. Saunders Co., 1981.

39. Schwartz, S., et al. Principles of Surgery, 4th ed. New York: McGraw-Hill Book Co., 1984.

40. Seifert, P. Mitral Valve Replacement. AORN Journal, Dec. 1982, pp. 959-972

41. Simmons, S. and Given, B. Nissen Fundoplication for Hiatus Hernia Repair. AORN Journal, July 1981, pp. 35-46.

42. Soloman, E. and Davis, P. Understanding Human Anatomy and Physiology. New York: McGraw Hill Inc., 1978.

43. Thomas, C., (ed.). Taber's Cyclopedic Medical Dictionary, 14th ed. Philadelphia: F. A. Davis Co., 1981.

44. West, K. Surgical Wound Infections: Causes and Treatment. JORRI, Sept. 1983, pp. 9, 12-14.